Teaching the History of Medicine
at a Medical Center

The Henry E. Sigerist Supplements to the
Bulletin of the History of Medicine

New Series, no. 7
Editor: Lloyd G. Stevenson, M.D.

Henry E. Sigerist, recruited by William H. Welch to be director of the Johns Hopkins Institute of the History of Medicine, was the founder of the *Bulletin of the History of Medicine* and also of the first series of supplements, which extended from 1943 to 1951. It was Sigerist's resolve that the *Bulletin* should provide the organ not only of the Johns Hopkins Institute but also of the American Association for the History of Medicine, and to this day it subserves both functions. It is therefore eminently suitable that the new series should bear the founder's name and perpetuate his scholarly interests. These interests were so broad and so varied that the supplements will recognize no narrow limits in range of theme and will publish historical essays of greater scope than the *Bulletin* itself can accommodate. It is not too much to hope that in time the Sigerist supplements will help to extend the purview of medical history.

Other Books in the New Series

1. *Almost Persuaded: American Physicians and Compulsory Health Insurance, 1912–1920,* by Ronald L. Numbers
2. *William Harvey and His Age: The Professional and Social Context of the Discovery of the Circulation,* edited by Jerome J. Bylebyl
3. *The Clinical Training of Doctors: an Essay of 1793* by Philippe Pinel, edited and translated, with an introductory essay, by Dora B. Weiner
4. *Times, Places, and Persons: Aspects of the History of Epidemiology,* edited by Abraham Lilienfeld
5. *When the Twain Meet: The Rise of Western Medicine in Japan,* by John Z. Bowers
6. *A Celebration of Medical History: The Fiftieth Anniversary of The Johns Hopkins Institute of the History of Medicine and The Welch Medical Library,* edited by Lloyd G. Stevenson

Based upon a Symposium sponsored by
The Josiah Macy, Jr., Foundation
in cooperation with
The Johns Hopkins Institute of
the History of Medicine

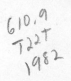

TEACHING THE HISTORY OF MEDICINE AT A MEDICAL CENTER

Edited by
Jerome J. Bylebyl

THE JOHNS HOPKINS UNIVERSITY PRESS
BALTIMORE AND LONDON

The Johns Hopkins University Press, Baltimore, Maryland 21218
The Johns Hopkins Press Ltd., London

Library of Congress Cataloging in Publication Data
Main entry under title:

Teaching the history of medicine at a medical
    center.

    (The Henry E. Sigerist supplements to the Bulletin
of the history of medicine; new ser., no. 7)
    Proceedings of a symposium sponsored by the
Josiah Macy, Jr. Foundation and the Johns Hopkins
University Institute of the History of Medicine.
    1. Medicine—History—Study and teaching—Congresses.
I. Bylebyl, Jerome J. II. Josiah Macy, Jr.
Foundation. III. Johns Hopkins University.
Institute of the History of Medicine. IV. Series.
R735.T4   610.9   82-148
ISBN 0-8018-2799-X   AACR2

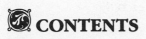 CONTENTS

Teaching the History of Medicine
at a Medical Center

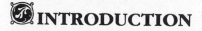INTRODUCTION

Jerome J. Bylebyl

This book is the offspring of a symposium held at the Johns Hopkins Medical School on 14 October 1980. It was organized by Lloyd G. Stevenson at the suggestion of John Z. Bowers, and was sponsored jointly by the Josiah Macy, Jr., Foundation and the Johns Hopkins Institute of the History of Medicine. There was wide agreement among those in attendance that the session was not only intellectually stimulating but also very useful in a nuts-and-bolts sort of way. It is therefore to be hoped that the published proceedings will be, if not an actual "how-to" manual, at least a source of practical strategies for those who either are currently involved in teaching medical history or are contemplating such a venture.

Appropriately, the symposium began with a broad view of the subject, followed by a variety of more specialized ones. The broad view was provided by Gert H. Brieger, who has had a wealth of experience teaching different kinds of students in the health professions at several leading centers. Based upon this experience, he sought to define the goals that ought to inform such teaching and advocated the adoption of the case study method as the best way to achieve these goals.

Most of the other presentations were also concerned with defining a role for history in the curricula of the health professions, but chiefly with reference to various other disciplines. Chester Burns addressed himself to the recent proliferation of programs in the medical humanities and suggested that it is in this context that the history of medicine may yet find its most useful and congenial place in the medical curriculum. Russell Maulitz also proposed a redefinition of disciplinary relationships, but along somewhat different lines. In his view, the history of medicine should undergo a metamorphosis from the long and narrow (Western medicine since antiquity), to the short and wide (the medicine of all cultures in the twentieth century), and, in the process, medical historians should strengthen their ties with medical anthropologists and sociologists. In contrast, Arthur Viseltear saw little need to abandon the long view of Western medicine since antiquity but argued that this focus on the past should be accompanied by a focus on the present through the involvement of the medical historian in the analysis of con-

1

temporary health policy issues. Again, Pauline Mazumdar was concerned with shifting the focus of medical history, but in relation to the parent discipline of general history. There has been, she noted, a recent marked growth among general historians of social history at the expense of intellectual history, and she argued that it is high time for medical historians to follow this trend not only in their research (as has already occurred), but in their teaching as well. Finally, John Parascandola drew our attention to the history of pharmacy, though as an autonomous discipline with its own long tradition of teaching and research, rather than as a potential hybridization partner for the history of medicine.

There was, then, a considerable variety of outlooks represented in the symposium, and the diversity was at least doubled by the provision of appropriate commentators on each of the main speakers: Guenter Risse on Brieger, Todd Savitt on Burns, Robert Hudson on Maulitz, Barbara Rosenkrantz on Viseltear, Edward Atwater on Mazumdar, and John Crellin on Parascandola. Completing the program were two additional presentations. The first was a thoroughly practical demonstration by Robert Joy on how to make effective use of slides in lectures on the history of medicine. The second was a thoroughly delightful reminiscence by Saul Jarcho on his own experiences with seminars in the history of medicine over a stretch of fifty years.

Although Dr. Jarcho's was the only presentation that was avowedly descriptive in character, it turned out that most of the speakers and commentators also included frank descriptions of what is being done at their institutions, and with what results. Moreover, since this natural history of the history of medicine contributed significantly to the practicality of the symposium mentioned above, it seemed appropriate to round it off in the present volume with three additional descriptive essays relating to situations not covered in the original proceedings. One of these is by Don Bates, and relates how an old program at an even older medical school has recently been transformed by the adoption of a cross-disciplinary approach. The other two essays, one by Col. Joy and the other by Alvin Rodin and Robert Reece, describe two very different approaches to teaching the history of medicine taken at two very new American medical schools. Dr. Stevenson has provided commentary on all three of these additional essays.

Thus, what follows is a combination of rationalism and empiricism, of description of what has been and is being done, together with suggestions for new departures as yet untried. This mixture will, I think, prove to be valuable to those who pick up this book in search of practical information and advice on how to begin or improve a program in medical history, although such readers may also be initially overwhelmed by the sheer diversity of the approaches and prescriptions that follow—a diversity that accurately mirrors the current state of medical history as an academic discipline. Indeed, although most of the contributors to this volume are recognized figures in the history of medicine, no two of them come from academic units bearing exactly the same designation. To be sure, three of them are affiliated with programs called, simply enough, "History of Medicine," but even these are differentiated as a "department," an "institute," and a "section." The others are variously housed in programs called: "Military Medicine and History," "History of Health Sciences," "History of Pharmacy," "History of Science," "History and Sociology of Science," "History and Philosophy of Science and Technology," "Medical Humanities," "Humanities and Social Studies in Medicine," "Medicine and Society," "Community Health Sciences," and "Community Health and Family Medicine." Thus, the history of medicine seems to be remarkably adaptive (some might say promiscuous) in its cohabitations, setting up house not only with various branches of practical medicine but also with the humanities, the social sciences, and the natural sciences, in addition to an occasional solitary life style.

Not surprising in view of this array of disciplinary affiliations is the great variety of approaches to teaching the history of medicine described and recommended in the following essays. The contributors reflect some basic disagreements regarding such questions as: Should the history of medicine be part of the required curriculum, or an elective subject? Should it be taught through lectures, or through a discussion format? What are the relative values of films and slides as teaching aids? Should the course attempt to survey the whole evolution of medicine from ancient to modern times, or should it focus primarily on recent developments? Alternatively, should it follow the case-study method of dealing with selected topics from various periods in some depth? Should primary attention be given to the social history of medicine, or to the development of medical theories and practices? Should the history of medicine be taught for its own sake, or as a means to elucidate various philosophical and practical problems in contemporary health care? Again, should it be approached as a subject in its own right, or freely intermingled with various other disciplines in the humanities and social sciences? Should it be taught by professionally qualified medical historians, or by interested persons drawn from elsewhere in the faculty? Finally, can the history of medicine be profitably taught to medical students at all?

Perhaps more perplexing than this plethora of ways to teach the history of medicine (or not to teach it, in some instances) is the way in which the various authors are spread clear across the spectrum from gloomy pessimism to glowing optimism with regard to the possibility of arousing serious interest in history within a medical center, especially among medical students. At one end of the scale are two contributors who express frank discouragement about the results of their efforts to stimulate interest in their own schools. Only slightly more hopeful are several authors who suggest that medical historians will have to change their approach in one of a variety of ways if they are to gain (or regain) a degree of acceptance that they do not now currently enjoy. Occupying the middle ground are a number of contributors who simply describe the approaches that they are now taking, and who express varying degrees of satisfaction regarding the outcome. Finally, to counterbalance the Jeremiahs, there is one author who is quite sanguine about what has been achieved at his own institution as well as about the possibility of making similar headway elsewhere.

Despite this great diversity of views regarding both the approaches to and the prospects of the history of medicine, there does run through most of the contributions to this volume an important common theme. It is, simply, that the history of medicine is peculiarly dependent upon local conditions. This does not mean that there are no good intrinsic reasons for teaching the history of medicine to students in the health professions, but that these reasons do not compel universal assent, especially in the face of limitations of financial resources and curricular time. Consequently, local perceptions are all-important in determining whether the subject is to exist at all, what will be its base within the institution, how it will be taught, and, ultimately, how well it will flourish.

Some examples drawn from the institutions represented in this volume will illustrate these points. The Yale Medical School has one of the strongest traditions of support for the history of medicine, stemming in large measure from the personal enthusiasm and influence of John Fulton and, less directly, of Harvey Cushing. These commitments were made concrete in 1939 with the decision to establish the Yale Medical Historical Library, and in 1960 with the inauguration of the Department of the History of Science and Medicine. This department soon gained an international reputation as one of the leading centers of graduate teaching and research, although these achievements did not make enough of a local impression to prevent the department from being formally dissolved in 1975. This closely coincided with the death of the incumbent of the chair of the history of medicine, and resulted in a period of uncertainty concerning the very existence of the subject at Yale. But owing largely to spontaneous expressions of support from within the medical faculty, this brief hiatus was ended by the decision to establish the new Section of the History of Medicine, to which two full-time faculty members have now been named. These are both tenured appointments, so the Yale Medical School has unequivocally reaffirmed its medical historical tradition with a major commitment of resources.

Yale has been somewhat less generous toward the history of medicine with regard to that other precious commodity, curricular time, as we learn from Professor Arthur Viseltear in his contribution to this volume. Still, the nine hours given to the subject are nine more than it has at the vast majority of medical schools. Furthermore, Viseltear relates that although his recent proposal to increase the number of hours to eighteen was turned down, it was met by a counterproposal from the curriculum committee to add nine hours on "History, Politics, and the Policy of Health," based upon a course that he has been giving in another context. Thus, although Viseltear does not now have the kind of expansion that he asked for, he nevertheless does have eighteen hours. And I, for one, can think of few more positive developments for our field than that a course whose title contains the word "history" should spontaneously be mandated by a medical school curriculum committee on the grounds that it is "necessary" for all medical students.

The Yale Medical School thus provides an example of where the history of medicine has long had and continues to have an unusually congenial home; for at least a partial contrast, I shall turn to the University of Toronto, whose representative has given one of the most pessimistic reports that follow. At Toronto, a new professorship of the history of medicine was established at about the same time as the new appointments were made at Yale, but under quite a different set of local circumstances. First, there was little previous tradition of formal activity in the history of medicine within the medical faculty at Toronto. And second, the initiative for establishing the chair came from outside the medical faculty, indeed from outside the university. It was the result of a decision by the late Jason Hannah to devote a substantial part of the resources of the Associated Medical Services to supporting a chair in the history of medicine at each of the five medical schools in the province of Ontario. Bearing out my thesis about the importance of local conditions, the responses to this differed considerably at the various schools. For example, the University of Western Ontario already had a strong local tradition of medical history, and so, not surprisingly, Western was first off the mark in filling their Hannah Chair. Again, at McMaster, a new and self-consciously innovative medical school, the possibility of adding a medical historian to the faculty was greeted with unmistakable enthusiasm, although it took several years before a suitable candidate could be found.

The Hannah seed has by no means fallen on barren soil at the University of Toronto, whose arts faculty has for some time included a strong institute of the history of science and technology. A historian of medicine was a natural addition to this group, and Pauline Mazumdar, Toronto's Hannah Professor, describes a vigorous program of undergraduate and graduate teaching that has already developed in this context. But, by Dr. Mazumdar's account, her reception within the medical school, especially among the medical students, has been decidedly underwhelming. Indeed, with regard to the specific theme of "teaching the history of medicine at a medical center," she all but advocates giving up the effort as hopeless. I would suggest, however, that generalizing from the particular conditions at Toronto to all medical schools and medical students would be unwarranted, and even the pessimism about Toronto may be somewhat premature. For in spite of all, some medical students have elected to take Dr. Mazumdar's course, and by focusing on the needs and interests of such students it may yet prove possible to nurture these slender beginnings into a new local tradition.

Thus, in stressing the importance of local conditions in sustaining the history of medicine, I do not mean to suggest that the subject is doomed to failure at schools that do not have a long-standing commitment to it. Traditions must have a beginning as well as a continuation, and there is no reason why that beginning must have occurred fifty years ago. In fact, in one of the essays by Col. Joy, we are provided with a glimpse of what will probably turn out to be a vigorous new local tradition at its very inception. Joy has entitled his essay "Starting from Scratch," though he might also have called it, "Starting a Tradition" or, even better, "Transplanting a Tradition," since his own interest in the history of medicine stems from his days as a medical student at Yale. Joy went on to a long and varied career in military medicine, whose most recent phase has been to participate in the planning and opening of the new armed forces medical school (USUHS). Having kept the faith through the years, he has seen to it that the history of medicine plays an important role in the new school. Indeed, at this, one of the newest medical schools in the country, the number of required hours in the history of medicine is, I believe, the largest of all.

It might be objected that this school is quite atypical, or that the history of medicine might have been disregarded even here, but for the fact that Col. Joy happened to be a medical historian in addition to being an influential figure on other grounds. However, my point is precisely that all medical schools are unique in certain important respects, and that support or lack of support for the history of medicine is one of the ways in which they reveal their individuality. Moreover, in those schools where the subject has become especially well established, it is usually because a particular individual who had more or less influence in the school happened also to be historically minded: Welch at Hopkins, Fulton at Yale, Middleton at Wisconsin, Wangensteen at Minnesota, Clendening at Kansas, or Saunders at San Francisco. I should add, though, that more than individual caprice is involved, because a significant number of these and other programs have now long survived the passing of their special patrons. Thus, it may be that where medical history has never existed, its absence is not sorely felt, but where it has once existed, its continuing presence seems to be at least tolerated and even appreciated.

In this respect, the history of medicine is markedly different from a subject such as physiology, whose inclusion in the medical curriculum is a matter of international rather than local consensus. Furthermore, the contents and methods of the physiology courses in different schools will also reflect the high degree of internal consensus that characterizes most of the natural sciences, but not the humanities or the social sciences. Parenthetically, one might note that less than a century ago physiology as presently conceived was to be found at only a handful of American medical schools, where its existence, also, could best be explained in terms of peculiar sets of local conditions and personalities. But it would be unrealistic to expect that the history of medicine will soon, if ever, reach a stage where, like physiology, its presence in the curriculum is the result of general standards rather than of particular circumstances.

Thus, teachers and would-be teachers of the subject will have to be flexible in adapting to a great variety of local environments, as well as resourceful in seeking to carve out new niches where they do not presently exist. I believe that their greatest asset in this endeavor will be the inherent fascination that the medicine of the past can have for those who are immersed in learning the medicine of the present and in creating the medicine of the future. Their greatest difficulty will be that of obtaining an initial hearing from students and health professionals whose time and attention spans are already filled close to, or even beyond, capacity. The strategy of finding some room in such a plenum will of necessity be inseparable from that of choosing the kind of medical history with which to fill it—some kinds will slip in more easily than others—but there are also ways of adding lubricity where it is not naturally present. Both choices will require careful consideration of the locally prevailing conditions as well as of the interests and style of the person or persons involved.

It is for this reason that the present volume, with its great diversity of approaches and institutional contexts, will probably prove to be of greater value than a single set of precepts on how to teach and what to teach. Consensus on these questions does not exist among those who currently teach the history of medicine, so any attempt to lay down a single set of norms would be arbitrary and possibly counterproductive. On the other hand, to say simply that "anything goes" as long as it passes for medical history among a certain local clientele would be equally misleading, since it would imply a complete lack of standards in a field that does, in fact, have a long tradition of competent scholarship and teaching. This collection of essays avoids both extremes by accurately mirroring the diversity of approaches that currently exists among those who represent the professionally qualified mainstream of the history of medicine. It may not provide ready-made solutions to the problems that are inherent in the teaching of our subject to students in medicine and the other health professions, but I believe that it will nevertheless prove quite useful to those who treat it as a source of raw materials out of which to create solutions that are appropriate to their particular local environments.

In keeping with this belief, I shall conclude this introduction by adding one more description of how the history of medicine is taught at a particular school, namely, at Johns Hopkins, where the local medical-historical tradition is one of the strongest in the country. Indeed, long before the Hopkins medical institutions were even opened, formal teaching in a medically related subject began at the university in 1877 with a course of lectures on the history of medicine by John Shaw Billings, who was at that time heavily involved in planning the hospital and medical school. In 1890, a year after the opening of the hospital and three years before the opening of the medical school, there was organized the Johns Hopkins Medical History Club, which recently observed its ninetieth anniversary. The leading spirit of the club at its inception was William Osler, who also wrote and published widely on medical-historical themes—an example that continues to be followed right up to the present by clinicians and basic scientists on the medical school faculty.

In 1928, an important new dimension was added with the inauguration of the Johns Hopkins Institute of the History of Medicine. William H. Welch, the elder statesman of medicine—not only at Hopkins but across the nation—was responsible for securing the financial support of the Rockefeller Foundation for this undertaking, which he hoped would serve as a counterweight to the scientific orientation of medicine that he had earlier done so much to bring about. Welch himself served briefly in the new professorship that was named after him, but perhaps his most important accomplishment in that capacity was to secure the services of a successor in the person of Henry Sigerist, who came to Hopkins from the Institute of the History of Medicine at Leipzig. Sigerist and his successors—Shryock, Temkin, and Stevenson—have established and maintained the institute as an international center of research and graduate training; indeed, seven of the contributors to this volume hold advanced degrees from the Hopkins Institute.

The teaching of medical students has also been a long-standing part of the institute's program, and since 1958, a course in the history of medicine has been a required part of the medical curriculum. Over the years, the number of hours allotted to this course has fluctuated considerably, from fifty to fourteen, and is currently set at eighteen. Three years ago, I was given responsibility for a complete revision of this course, so that in its present state it is essentially a new course that is still at the shakedown stage. I had had no previous involvement with a course that was expressly intended for medical students, although I believe that my lack of experience was balanced by a change in the curriculum that gave me a significant advantage over my immediate predecessor. Previously, the course was situated at the beginning of the first year of medical studies, a time when the students feel all the pressures of adapting to the new world of the medical school and when they as yet know relatively little about medicine as distinct from the general biology of their premedical years. Thus, one had to try to introduce them to the history of something—medicine—that was itself still rather alien to them both socially and intellectually. However, my assumption of responsibility for the course coincided with its shift to the beginning of the second year, when the students seem to be better suited to make sense of the subject: they have had a full year of exposure to the medical environment, they are immersed in the study of pathology, and they are undergoing their first introduction to clinical skills.

As I shall indicate, this new location of the history of medicine within the curriculum had a significant influence on the design of the course, but a number of other considerations were also important. First, there was the fact that the course is required: all the medical students must take the course, and they must receive a passing grade if they are to be awarded their medical degrees. Most of my previous experience had been with teaching elective courses and seminars, where the teacher has considerable leeway to design the course as he sees fit because the students can choose not to take the course if they see fit. However, I find myself in agreement with the view expressed below by Col. Joy that making a course required puts restrictions on the teacher as well as on the students. That is, most required courses in the medical curriculum are intended to provide a comprehensive introduction to a particular subject, rather than to expose the student to selected aspects of it. Accordingly, many students will naturally approach a course in the history of medicine with the expectation that it will fulfill such a goal, and, I believe, they would be quite justified in feeling cheated if the course did not cover what they regarded as the basic essentials.

On the other hand, if one were to try to give a truly comprehensive survey of the history of medicine in the space of eighteen one-hour lectures, it would almost certainly turn out to be the proverbial litany of names, discoveries, and dates that give the term "survey course" a deservedly bad reputation. It would also conflict with another basic requirement, namely, that the lectures must be of sufficient interest to induce the students to attend, since making a course required is no guarantee that this will happen. Therefore, rather than trying to pack the whole history of medicine into eighteen hours, I set out to try to define eighteen topics, each of which could be dealt with in a single self-contained lecture, and which would, in the aggregate, cut a fairly broad swath through the traditional mainstream of the history of medicine. However, I would make no attempt to touch all bases through summary and enumeration; either a topic would be included as a major lecture topic or it would not be included at all.

Another question that I had to consider was that of "relevance," that is, whether and to what extent the historical lectures should serve as a forum for commenting on current issues in medicine. Fortunately, local conditions made it relatively easy to reach a decision in this regard; the Hopkins medical students have during their first year a course of more than fifty hours on current ethical and social issues in medicine. Thus, there was no need to try to make the history of medicine do double service in this regard, although this did not mean that I conceived of the course as having no relationship to current issues. On the contrary, I made it a point to familiarize myself with the content of the issues course, and this made it possible to allude to these matters at appropriate points in the historical lectures without having to enter very far into the substance of the contemporary debates.

Finally, as mentioned above, the overall focus of the course was also influenced by its new location within the curriculum. As noted, the course is now given at a time when the students are primarily immersed in the study of pathology. Indeed, the history of medicine is quite literally surrounded by disease: the lectures, given on Tuesdays and Thursdays at noon, are preceded by three hours of pathology and followed (after a lunch break) by three hours of pathophysiology. Accordingly, without turning the course into a history of pathology, I decided to give special emphasis to the development of ideas about disease, especially to the various ways in which disease has been made the object of scientific investigation from the seventeenth to the twentieth centuries.

But while the main focus of the course would thus be the development of scientific medicine in the modern era, with the greatest weight given to the nineteenth century, I was not prepared to neglect completely the medicine of other periods and cultures, because I believe that a comparative perspective is essential for an understanding of modern medicine. Five introductory lectures are intended to provide these elements. The first is entitled "Disease and Culture," and deals with two broad themes: the role of cultural evolution as the prime determinant of the health of the human population, and the role of culture as the screen through which disease is consciously perceived and experienced by a given society. The second considers the phenomenon of medical practices as widespread but problematic facets of human behavior. It includes some films of traditional practitioners at work in various parts of the world.

The third lecture is on Hippocratic medicine, and seeks to provide an overview of the medical practitioners and practices of the fifth and fourth centuries B.C. within the context of contemporary Greek society and culture. The following lecture is entitled "Physicians and Surgeons," and is concerned primarily with the emergence of a stratified medical profession in medieval Europe and with the eventual unification of the profession in more recent centuries. The fifth lecture is devoted to the growth of anatomy as the first major area of systematic empirical research that is related to medicine. Attention is given to such issues as religious and social barriers to the dissection of the human body, and the importance of anatomical research as an area of common ground between physicians and surgeons and as a source of professional prestige for both.

The remaining topics then follow in a fairly straightforward manner, and need no detailed commentary: the discovery of the circulation; the study of disease from Sydenham to Morgagni; the Paris clinical school; epidemiology and public health in the nineteenth century; the emergence of the full-time medical scientist in Europe; Virchow and cellular pathology; bacteriology; the American medical profession; medicine at Johns Hopkins; the development of modern surgery (given by Peter Olch); twentieth century clinical research (given by A. McGehee Harvey); and therapeutics in the twentieth century, especially the introduction of antibiotics.

Except for the two guest lectures, all of the sessions are slide lectures, that is, they are accompanied throughout by a continuous series of slides rather than being occasionally illustrated by them. During the past two years, funds from the university's Human Biology Program, which is based on an overall grant from the Commonwealth Fund, have made it possible for our institute to acquire about four thousand new slides, intended to serve as a long-term teaching resource as well as to be used for this particular course. The slides are of charts and important quotations as well as of pictures and objects, so their use does not necessarily restrict the subject matter to things that are inherently visual. It has been my experience that they can help to make a lecture not only more effective but also more efficient, in the sense that one can cover more ground with a combination of words and images than with words alone, an important consideration when curricular time is limited. The required readings for the course include photocopies of articles and excerpts from primary sources that are handed out at most of the lectures, as well as a book—Donald Fleming's *William H. Welch and the*

Rise of Modern Medicine—which is available at the bookstore. The students may choose between a final exam and a term paper as the basis of their grade (the majority prefer the exam).

To conclude, I shall cite the major results of a student questionnaire conducted at the end of the course last fall (1981). I do so with some hesitation because it is difficult to know how to evaluate the results in the absence of comparative data. In the essays and comments that follow in this book, however, fairly numerous references are made to medical students and their attitudes toward the history of medicine, so I thought that it might be useful to have at least some quantitative data in this regard, even if it pertains to only one particular course in one particular year at one particular school. Ninety-eight out of 117 students completed the survey, with the following (partial) results:

Scale: 1 = Unsatisfactory, weak, etc.; 2 = Below average; 3 = Average, satisfactory; 4 = Above average, very good; 5 = Excellent, outstanding; N = No opinion.

	1	2	3	4	5	N
General significance of subject	2%	4%	28%	47%	18%	1%
Scope and orientation of this course	0	3	21	60	14	1
Adequacy of execution	0	5	38	44	12	1
Was it rewarding, useful to you?	1	7	28	45	18	1
Rating of slides	0	2	23	42	29	4
Overall evaluation of course	1	1	32	56	9	1

I understand that these ratings compare favorably with those of other courses in the second year curriculum, and believe that these and other qualitative indications of student reaction justify at least a negative conclusion: the would-be teacher of the history of medicine need not be overly concerned as to the inherent palatability of the subject for medical students.

THE HISTORY OF HEALTH AND DISEASE FOR HEALTH PROFESSIONALS: THE CASE STUDY APPROACH

Gert H. Brieger

I. Much has been written about the place of medical history in the curriculum. George Rosen's long summary needs no repetition here.[1] Nor do we need to say much about the utility of medical history, the subject of a conference at the New York Academy of Medicine in 1957.[2] A Macy-sponsored conference at the National Library of Medicine in 1966 addressed such questions as "What Medical History Should be Taught to Medical Students," "Who Should Teach the History of Medicine," and "How to Support and Promote the History of Medicine." The resulting small monograph, edited by John Blake, published in 1968 is readily available.[3] More recently, Lester King edited an able symposium in *Clio Medica* with articles by Chester Burns, Guenter Risse, Robert Hudson, and others.[4]

Our field has not lacked for surveys either. Chester Burns has neatly summed up the six or so surveys about the teaching of medical history beginning with one originated by Eugene Cordell here in Baltimore at the beginning of the century, and the most recent and most extensive one carried out by Genevieve Miller at the end of the 1960s.[5] I have briefly summarized all this in a section of a long chapter on the history of medicine just recently published in a book entitled *A Guide to the Culture of Science, Technology, and Medicine.*[6] Surely, enough is enough!

While I have refrained until now from writing about teaching strategies for the history of the health sciences, I have thought about it a great deal. When I stop to count the different types of students I have encountered and the various settings in which I have taught, or in which I believed I was teaching, I realize that my experiences are probably as wide and varied as anyone's. I list these only to show you my perspective—or, as they like to say in California, to "show you where I'm coming from."

I have taught (and I use the term loosely and with much hesitation) in three schools of medicine, two schools of public health, on three college campuses in both undergraduate as well as graduate courses, in continuing education, and in summer seminars. Since going to a health science campus in San Francisco, I have actually seen more students from the schools of nursing and pharmacy than I have from the school of medicine. What these experiences have "taught" me—that is, what I am now able to see much more clearly than I saw even five years ago— is a fairly profound sense of skepticism about much of the so-called teaching I have attempted. There probably is no "right" way or "best" way to teach history to medical center students. But I have come to some conclusions about a wrong way.

For fifteen years I have participated in or run courses that for lack of a better designation may be called survey courses in the history of medicine. I plan to stop teaching this kind of course for professional school students, despite the fact they often are fairly well received. I have now slowly but surely come to believe that they are intellectually too often at a very superficial level, and that the survey, while it may be entertaining, is not terribly enlightening and is therefore probably a waste of time for those students who are as tightly scheduled as are medical and other health science students.

I will not deny that a survey course in the history of medicine, from Imhotep to whatever grand figure of the 1970s you might wish to name, has a place on the college campus, as does, for instance, "Western Civilization." I believe that a good survey course must be accompanied by a fair amount of reading, and it should be followed by further, more focused courses in the history of medicine. Medical students, in my experience at least, who elect history courses, do so because they are interested in broadening their understanding of their profession. Usu- ally they are not burning to read much, nor usually do they have the time to do so. Furthermore, most health professional students do well if they can take one history course, so they do not have time for history 168 and 175 that follow history 4A and B, as is the case on the college campus.

Lest I be accused of having declared God is dead, or having styled myself the Ivan Illich of medical history—he who merely criticizes but offers no solutions—I would like to say something about what I believe we should be doing. I realize that brevity makes me out to be unduly provocative, but such is the lot of the lead-off batter.

I have said nothing about justifying the history of medicine, either to a curriculum committee or to our students. Much has been written about this and we do not, in 1980 in Baltimore, have to repeat it. Let me just note in passing that I believe the question, "What do we learn from history?" is wrongly phrased. It is from trying to learn about history, from the efforts required to achieve an historical perspective, that we may learn about how people as individuals or in groups solved the problems of meeting their common human needs. It is a process of thinking, then, that may have value, a process of criticism, of the posing of questions; it is the imaginative approach itself, that needs to be learned. Merely giving students a series of historical facts is much like giving them anatomy without physiology.

Medicine is itself an eminently historical endeavor. There is history *in* medicine as well as history *of* medicine.[7] The first thing a young student is taught in the clinical setting is to take a history. Ward rounds are a series of clinical histories. The CPC is a historical exercise. Ultimately, it is the task of the physician, as indeed it is also that of the historian, to gather evidence, to make decisions about its validity or its degree of certainty, to make judgments regarding diagnoses, treatment, and if possible, in that best of all worlds, prevention.

It is the development of those critical faculties that medical education should foster in order to prepare students for a career as decision makers. It is here, that the history of medicine in its broadest sense may be no more or no less useful than any other disciplined way of thinking and problem solving.

Nearly ten years ago Dr. Stevenson and I participated in some very pleasant festivities celebrating the opening of a new health science library at the University of North Carolina in Chapel Hill. I defended, at that time, my right to pursue medical history for its own sake, but I also, on the opposite pole defended the instrumentalist approach to history. So popular among historians of the Progressive Era, instrumentalism referred to the conscious use of history to aid in the solution of problems. Contemporary history, of which so many historians are skeptical, is of increasing interest and potential on health science campuses. It is a truism, as Roy MacLeod has recently written of the history of science, that today much historiography reflects contemporary concerns.[8] Rightly or wrongly, whether we like it or not, that is the view of most health professional students and of most of our colleagues on medical center faculties. All this is a subject for an entire conference, so suffice it to say, if that is the game, let us play it.

The teaching strategy that I believe makes the most sense is one I am a novice in developing for myself, but it is one that our colleagues in schools of law and of business have used for over a century: the case method. Some teachers of the history of health sciences have also used this approach for a long time. I realize that I am not proposing anything really new or revolutionary. I have seen course outlines from Yale, the University of Wisconsin, Cincinnati, and Rochester, to name but a few, that in part, at least, embody the case method. At the Madison meeting of the American Association for the History of Medicine, Guenter Risse arranged a marvelous example of a case study for a symposium: the swine flu vaccine story. It has appeared as a book edited by June Osborn.[9] This episode has received enough attention from historians, virologists, and political scientists, that a sizeable body of literature is available.[10] It is an example of the usefulness of history, in this case contemporary history, to assist in the formulation of health policy.

Judith Swazey and Karen Reeds have recently published a series of case studies in a book entitled *Today's Medicine, Tomorrow's Science,* wherein they elucidate ways in which categorical or disease-oriented research has contributed to the understanding of fundamental biological phenomena.[11] And so the literature grows. I will make no attempt to review it all here.

II. I am not entirely happy with the designation "case method" for what I am advocating, but for lack of a better term, I will use it for now. At any rate, I have become convinced that we ought to listen to our medical students who complain that they are deluged with facts, that little is done to make what they are forced to learn have meaning in a larger sense, and that there is insufficient problem solving in their education, especially in the preclinical years. I have become equally convinced that by means of specific, concrete examples we can communicate a sense of historical perspective that entails an active rather than a passive method of learning, and that, above all, will engage students with problems that have a real meaning for them.

In the winter of 1900 a twenty-nine-year-old fourth-year medical student at Harvard, Walter B. Cannon, wrote an eloquent plea for the use of "The Case Method of Teaching Systematic Medicine." Published as a five and a half page article in the *Boston Medical and Surgical Journal,* Cannon's piece described the rising dissatisfaction with the usual method of teaching by didactic lectures. Cannon claimed that it was not an economical use of the students' time, that it allowed for a slighting of studies during the term and favored cramming at the end, and, most importantly, that it was an inefficient means for developing mental training for medical work. "Why, then," Cannon asked, "should medical students be expected to reason clearly in medical matters, weigh conflicting evidence or draw just conclusions, when their chief practice is taking lecture notes?" [12]

Cannon acknowledged that he was heavily influenced by what he knew was going on in the classrooms of the Harvard Law School. Under the aegis of the dean, Christopher C. Langdell, the law school had since the 1870s been pioneering the case method approach to teaching. Cannon believed that for the practice of medicine the successful physician had to develop two skills: observation and interpretation. Observation gave data, and this data had to be properly explained and interpreted in order to make diagnoses and prognoses and give the proper treatment.

It was the development of these skills that the case method fostered so well.

In the history of science the best known examples of the case method approach are those developed by James B. Conant and Leonard K. Nash at Harvard. Of special interest to the history of the health sciences are those on Pasteur's study of fermentation and on Pasteur's and Tyndall's study of spontaneous generation. Larry Holmes, who had direct experience as an assistant in the Harvard course that used the case studies, has written a thoughtful chapter on their applicability for the history of medicine in Edwin Clarke's 1971 book on *Modern Methods*. [13] I do not need here to repeat the criticisms and advantages so well elucidated by Holmes.

In reading the common foreword to these case studies, it becomes very evident that what Conant had in mind was to bring to the non-scientist an "understanding" of science, of the methods used by the scientist to pose a question and to solve a problem. All citizens, Conant claimed, need to be aware of what science can or cannot accomplish if, as intelligent members of society, we are to make a whole series of policy decisions based upon such an understanding.

The same points may, of course, be made about medicine. I have long been interested in writing an updated version of Henry Sigerist's *Einfuhrung in die Medizin,* because I believe that it is one of the historian's tasks to introduce medicine. Such a course, or a course with this as a main emphasis, I have taught to college undergraduates both at Duke and in Berkeley. Here, more of a survey approach may still be quite appropriate, but a series of good case studies could be very useful to introduce the problems of medical science and medical practice.

My reasons for wishing to stress the case method for teaching health professional students the history of the broad field we call medicine are not merely to introduce facts or elucidate the evolution of ideas, but rather to illustrate, by means of historical examples, what medical problems arose, what their implications were for the health of society or for economic welfare—as well as for the welfare of the professionals who had to deal with these phenomena.

In thinking about restructuring my courses away from the survey or topical-lecture format toward either discussions and more thorough analyses of the development of certain ideas or practices, or the use of specific trends or events as "cases" for study, I have been influenced by those who have had much more experience in these matters than I. A very provocative example of what I am trying to do for the history of the health sciences may be seen in Ernest R. May's little book *"Lessons" of the Past: The Use and Misuse of History in American Foreign Policy* (1973). [14] Using policy questions facing the United States government at

the end of World War II, in the Korean War, and again during the 1960s
in Vietnam, Professor May brings clearly into focus how policy makers
used, did not use, or actually misused history. In his preface, May tells
his readers that the book has three theses:

1. That framers of foreign policy are often influenced by beliefs about what
   history teaches or portends;
2. That policy makers ordinarily use history badly;
3. And, that policy makers can, if they will, use history in a more discrimi-
   nating manner.

While our courses in history that we generally offer in medical
centers need not be aimed primarily at policy makers, they surely do
touch those people who will be making all kinds of decisions—some
very technical, some of a psychological or philosophical nature—and
surely they will make hundreds of decisions, on either a macro- or a
micro-scale, that will have profound social and economic consequences. My task here is not to justify a place for medical history but to
begin the discussion of how best to communicate what we like to call a
historical perspective or a historical awareness to a group of action-
oriented students. We should not waste our time here, nor in our
classrooms I believe, justifying or defending the place of medical history
in the medical curriculum. It has been ably defended by our predecessors who were, actually, more eloquent than I am able to be. The task
before us now is to illustrate for students the "uses" and abuses of
history.

III. I do not have the time here to discuss the weaknesses inherent
in the case method approach to teaching. Nor can I elaborate on a
related subject about which I hope to write something, namely, the
importance of the medical historian becoming involved in writing contemporary history. Obviously, if one chooses cases such as the swine flu
vaccine, that is precisely what one does. Surely Arthur Viseltear has set a
very high standard for us to follow.[15]

I wish, instead, to give a few examples of issues, trends, or events
that I believe will make very interesting case studies. I have heard Professor May describe the course that he and Richard Neustadt teach at the
Kennedy School at Harvard. Each of the cases they developed required
a minimum of 200 hours to prepare properly. Is it any wonder that most
of us take the easy way out and sit down for an hour or two and write
out notes for a lecture?

I will limit myself to giving you, briefly, a few examples of cases I
am presently preparing. I am only in the first few hours of the long process. I will mention only the bare outline of these cases, not describing
the varieties of historical directions in which they may be followed.

Because of my own interests in the history of surgery as well as in the phenomenon of acceptance of medical innovation or resistance to change, I have long been intrigued by the story of the surgical treatment of mitral stenosis. Lauder Brunton, a British cardiologist of note, first suggested a possible surgical cure as early as 1902.[16] While some work was done in France, it was not until the 1920s that a few patients were operated upon. One reason usually given for the long delay is that the prevailing cardiological views of James MacKenzie were opposed to surgery because he believed the disease was fundamentally one of myocardium rather than endocardium. Thus the first intriguing issue illustrated by this example is the role of the "influential" in either spreading or retarding a medical practice. The role of outspoken, self-assured physicians, often older and well established, whom we might refer to as medical mandarins, needs much more exploration.

After a series of cases reported by Elliot Cutler and Samuel Levine in the 1920s, not until the late 1940s was the procedure again pursued. It is true that Cutler's results were very poor, yet Henry Souttar in England had one highly successful case in 1925.

Judith Swazey and Renee Fox have written an interesting paper about all this, exploring the story of a clinical moratorium in terms of the experiment versus therapy dilemma, the dual role of the physician as healer and as investigator, and the influence of lay opinion and cultural conceptions and beliefs.[17] More is to be done with the history of mitral valve surgery itself. Obviously the students will have to read some of the literature and suffer along with those who worked to develop mitral commissurotomy as a useful and effective method of therapy.[18]

Another surgical practice with which every present-day medical and nursing student is very familiar is early ambulation after surgery or childbirth. Without even trying to be systematic, I have collected from the American literature between 1941 and 1954 over fifty articles and one book on the subject.[19] Early ambulation, or early rising as it is frequently called, was used and defended by surgeons, gynecologists, and obstetricians who observed that the total period of convalescence was shortened, postoperative complications were markedly reduced, and the spirit of patients much improved.

Many surgeons, if not most of them, kept patients in bed for two or three weeks after operation. In the early 1940s, it seems, they were quite unaware that a literature on the subject of early rising had begun to appear forty or more years earlier, at the turn of the century. With the exigencies of World War II upon hospitals, nurses, and physicians, early ambulation was rediscovered. Ephraim McDowell became a hero again because Jane Todd Crawford, who was up making her bed within five days, obviously had used early ambulation, not just blind luck.

Besides illustrating changing historical interpretations, this case illustrates a wide variety of interesting and important implications. First of all, as is illustrated by the mitral valve case, there was a moratorium in its use. Daniel J. Leithauser, a Detroit surgeon who was very active in popularizing the method in the early 1940s, wrote, "At the time I became interested in the problem, I did not know that 'early rising' had been practised by other surgeons." [20] Not an unusual occurrence in the history of medicine. Also there is a technical side to all this because sutures and anesthesia were improved between 1900 and 1940.

Leithauser suggests that the early work on the subject was of experimental interest only and did not become standard practice because it was reported by nonacademic surgeons. This obviously raises many interesting questions about so-called medical advances and where they were effectively made. So too, it relates to the phenomenon of the medical mandarins.

The economic implications for hospitals of the practice of up-and-out-of-bed are immense, and will lead the student of this case into many issues and developments about medical care and hospitals; and I have said nothing of the tremendous implications for military medicine.

Thus it is readily apparent, to me at least, that what at first glance sounds like a fairly narrow subject is indeed extremely broad and illustrative of not only the practice of medicine but also its administration, financing, and distribution.

A topic of central interest to medicine as well as of society today is the role of the hospital. Fortunately, at long last we are beginning to have, in works by Morris Vogel and Charles Rosenberg for instance, some good historical treatment of the place of hospitals in American medicine. One development or trend that may be used to elucidate much about hospitals, about medical practice, and about the costs of health care is found in the startling statistics of the numbers of hospitals. According to one survey, in 1873 there were 178 hospitals in this country, only 120 of which were general hospitals. Shortly after 1900 there were over 4000. This striking increase may serve as a provocative case study from which one may learn a great deal about the evolution of medical practice. [21]

Closely related to the numbers of hospitals is the whole notion of practice within them. A series of cases could be constructed around hospitals charts, as suggested by the Rockefeller Institute scientist A. R. Dochez in 1939. [22] He compared the charts of a patient with heart disease entering the hospital in 1910 with one who was treated in 1938. An even more startling difference would be seen if we used 1940 and 1980. One could do this for a variety of clinical conditions, prior to certain types of diagnostic procedures or therapeutic regimens and compare them to similar illness seen after the introduction of newer methods. Time in hospital, costs, nursing procedures, and a variety of other comparisons might easily be made. The use of real examples rather than abstract trends would be a useful pedagogical device, I believe.

Another example of a potential case study rich in its implications comes from the history of medical education. In 1925 virtually all applicants who had completed their premedical requirements were admitted to medical school, and according to one report the so-called Class A schools had an additional 1500 vacancies. In 1950, a mere twenty-five years later, in a time of decidedly higher or more stringent admission prerequisites, more than 24,000 students applied for just over 7000 places in the country's 79 medical schools. One out of 3.47 applicants was accepted that year. These figures are the more startling when one also considers that as late as 1940 only 1.5 million Americans (15 percent of their age group) went beyond high school in their education.[23]

This rather striking change in a quarter of a century, much like the case of the hospitals, raises many interesting questions about the medical profession in American society. Both case studies lend themselves to exploration of issues with which students may have a very personal sense of identification.

The final example will actually be the focus of an entire course in my department, but the idea of the right to health care may also provide any number of interesting case studies. Carleton Chapman's long article on the subject as it pertains to the history of medicine in America illustrates the many avenues one may follow.[24] But the idea of the right to health, besides having an interesting philosophical basis, may also be a convenient means of studying or comparing health care systems and the value of health in other cultures. One existing monograph that serves as a very fine example of a case study that pertains to this topic is Louis Cohn-Haft's work on the public physician in ancient Greece.[25]

Obviously brevity has caused me to leave out of the discussion the many possible questions these few examples might raise. I believe they will prove much more useful in providing for students what we like to call a historical perspective than will the usual survey of ancient, medieval, and Renaissance medicine, the accomplishments of the Paris School, the sanitary revolution, and so on. Obviously the discussion of any clinical case will lead us back to Bichat, Laennec, and Louis. What we want to do, after all, is to enlarge the student's horizon so that he or she will look up from their microscopes and textbooks to consider the importance of social structure as well as of cell structure.

Notes

1. George Rosen, "The place of history in medical education," *Bull. Hist. Med.*, 1948, *22:* 594–627; reprinted in Rosen's collection of essays, *From Medical Police to Social Medicine; Essays in the History of Health Care* (New York: Science History Publications, 1974), pp. 3–36. See also the very thoughtful paper by Owsei Temkin, "An essay on the usefulness of medical history for medicine," *Bull. Hist. Med.*, 1946, *19:* 9–47; reprinted in Temkin's *The Double Face of Janus and Other Essays in the History of Medicine* (Baltimore: The Johns Hopkins University Press, 1977), pp. 68–100.

2. Iago Galdston, ed., *On the Utility of Medical History* (New York: International Universities Press, 1957). See especially I. Galdston, "On the utility of medical history," pp. 3–9; G. Rosen, "Purposes and values of medical history," pp. 11–19; O. Temkin, "A critique of medical historiography," pp. 21–34; and E. Ackerknecht, "On the teaching of medical history," pp. 41–49.

3. John B. Blake, ed., *Education in the History of Medicine* (New York: Hafner, 1968).

4. *Clio Medica*, 1975, *10:* 129–65; 295–308.

5. Chester R. Burns, "History in medical education: the development of current trends in the United States," *Bull. N.Y. Acad. Med.*, 1975, *51:* 851–69. See also Guenter B. Risse, "Whither healing? The place of medical history in shaping the future role of medicine," *MD Magazine*, February 1979, pp. 9–11; Ilza Veith, "The function and place of the history of medicine in medical education," *J. Med. Ed.*, 1956, *31:* 303–9; F. F. Cartwright, "The place of medical history in undergraduate education," *Proc. Roy. Soc. Med.*, 1969, *62:* 1053–60; for a comparative view in a series of articles on teaching medical history in England, Switzerland, France, Spain, and Argentina, see *World Med. J.*, 1970, *17:* 49–64, and for a contentious and negative view with a thoughtful and witty rejoinder, see Iago Galdston, "On the futility of medical history," *Canad. Med. J.*, 1965, *93:* 807–11, and Lloyd G. Stevenson, "'Fortuitous genius' and the history of medicine," *Canad. Med. J.*, 1965, *93:* 874–77.

6. Gert H. Brieger, "History of medicine," ch. 3 in *A Guide to the Culture of Science, Technology, and Medicine*, ed. Paul T. Durbin (New York: Free Press, 1980), pp. 121–94.

7. The sociologists have written about this for their field. See especially Robert Straus, "The nature and status of medical sociology," *Amer. Sociol. Rev.*, 1957, *22:* 200–4.

8. Roy MacLeod, "Changing perspectives in the social history of science," ch. 5 in *Science, Technology and Society*, ed. Ina Spiegel-Rosing and Derek de Solla Price (Beverly Hills: Sage Publications, 1977), pp. 149–95; p. 149.

9. June E. Osborn, ed., *Influenza in America, 1918–1976* (New York: Prodist, 1977).

10. See, for example, Richard E. Neustadt and Harvey V. Fineberg, *The Swine Flu Affair: Decision-making on a Slippery Disease* (Washington, D.C.: U.S. Dept. HEW, 1978).

11. Judith P. Swazey and Karen Reeds, *Today's Medicine, Tomorrow's Science; Essays on Paths of Discovery in the Biomedical Sciences* (Washington, D.C.: U.S. Dept. HEW, 1978). Case studies included describe Pasteur's work, beriberi and vitamin B, sickle cell anemia and protein structure, and multiple myeloma and antibodies.

12. Walter B. Cannon, "The case method of teaching systematic medicine," *Boston Med. Surg. J.*, 1900, *142:* 31–36; p. 32.

13. Frederic L. Holmes, "The case history method in the historiography of medical sciences," ch. 12 in *Modern Methods in the History of Medicine*, ed. Edwin Clarke (London: Athlone Press, 1971), pp. 211–32. For one example in teaching the history of medicine see, Alvin E. Rodin and Alfonso J. Strano, "Case-oriented presentation of medical history: the D.E.A.D. conference," *J. Med. Educ.*, 1967, *42:* 886–91 (D.E.A.D. refers to Diagnostic Exercises on Ancient Disease).

14. Available as an Oxford University Press paperback edition.

15. See his essay, "A short political history of the 1976 swine influenza legislation," in Osborn, *Influenza in America*, pp. 29–58.

16. I have collected a very fat folder full of materials about the beginnings of mitral surgery. A convenient summary may be found in Stephen L. Johnson, *The History of Cardiac Surgery: 1896–1955* (Baltimore: The Johns Hopkins University Press, 1970), pp. 87–99. The elucidation of Sir James MacKenzie's role needs much further work, I believe.

17. Judith P. Swazey and Renee C. Fox, "The clinical moratorium: a case study of mitral valve surgery," in *Experimentation with Human Subjects*, ed. Paul A. Freund (New York: Braziller, 1970), pp. 315–57.

18. I am aware of the potential criticism to the effect that students studying this case may learn much about mitral valve surgery but hear nothing about Laennec's discovery of the stethoscope. My view of such teaching encompasses the development of our understanding of the diease as well as its diagnosis. Not only the invention of the stethoscope would become a part of the story, but the description of the murmur, the treatment of cardiac failure, as well as the surgical attempts to cure the disease of mitral stenosis would all have to be included in the full development of the case study. Obviously this is not one that would readily lend itself to a mere one-hour discussion.

19. See especially Daniel J. Leithauser, *Early Ambulation and Related Procedures in Surgical Management* (Springfield: Charles C Thomas, 1946). The articles and the book are primary sources. No historian has yet, to my knowledge, dealt with this important phenomenon.

20. Ibid., p. 10.

21. See J. M. Toner, "Statistics of regular medical associations and hospitals of the United States," *Trans. A.M.A.*, 1873, *24:* 287–333; Charles Rosenberg, "And heal the sick: the hospital and the patient in 19th century America," *J. Soc. Hist.*, 1977, *10:* 428–47; idem, "Inward vision and outward glance: the shaping of the American hospital, 1880–1914," *Bull. Hist. Med.*, 1979, *53:* 346–91; Morris Vogel, "Patrons, practitioners and patients: the voluntary hospital in mid–Victorian Boston," in *Victorian America,* ed. Daniel W. Howe (Philadelphia: University of Pennsylvania Press, 1976), pp. 121–38; idem, "Machine politics and medical care: the city hospital at the turn of the century," in *The Therapeutic Revolution,* ed. Morris J. Vogel and Charles E. Rosenberg (Philadelphia: University of Pennsylvania Press, 1979), pp. 159–75; and idem, *The Invention of the Modern Hospital: Boston 1870–1930* (Chicago: University of Chicago Press, 1980).

22. Alphonse R. Dochez, "President's address," *Trans. Amer. Clin. Climatol. Assoc.,* 1939, *53:* xviii–xxvi.

23. Aura E. Severinghaus, Harry J. Carman, and William E. Cadbury, *Preparation for Medical Education in the Liberal Arts College* (New York: McGraw-Hill, 1953), p. 19.

24. Carleton B. Chapman and John M. Talmadge, "The evolution of the right to health concept in the United States," *Pharos,* 1971, *34:* 30–51.

25. Louis Cohn-Haft, *The Public Physicians of Ancient Greece* (Northampton, Mass.: Smith College, Department of History, 1956).

⚜ COMMENTARY

Guenter B. Risse

⚜ I shall briefly comment on Dr. Brieger's suggestions and link them with remarks about my own teaching experience. In the first place, I must confess that I share his scepticism with regard to survey courses for future health professionals. Most of them are shallow, chronologically arranged catalogues of medical achievements lacking a clear focus and organization. At the University of Wisconsin Medical School this format was abandoned in 1971 due to student disinterest. The change in study plans was made easier since the required course had already been demoted to a minor elective during the 1968 curriculum reform and had not been taught for several years. The backbone of medico-historical teaching for over twenty years, this survey had endured numerous curricular revisions and remained virtually unchanged in content. In fact, after Erwin Ackerknecht's departure in 1957, our medical school specifically hired a number of German historians of medicine as visiting professors for one semester in order to have this course taught to the medical students.[1]

The new course, simply entitled "Historical Perspectives in Medicine," was based on the rationale that history could be employed as a tool to teach students how to assess contemporary problems critically in the light of past experiences and processes. Thus, in my opinion it was no longer necessary to present an extensive body of knowledge to be systematically mastered by the students through lectures and readings, but instead to select certain specific issues for thorough study and discussion in a seminar format. The word study must be emphasized, since I agree with Owsei Temkin that discussions cannot take place without a knowledge of the relevant historical facts.[2] Given the semester system in our school, fifteen topics were chosen with the help of students on the basis of instructor expertise, contemporary interest, and suitability for historical analysis.[3]

Therefore, I fully agree with Dr. Brieger's pedagogical objectives. The question, however, is how can we implement them? His single prescription is the employment of a case method using specific historical examples. Indeed, he wants to illustrate certain problems in medicine, and his examples refer to professional authoritarianism, the use and abuse of evidence, the role of faddism, as well as the economics and ethics of health care. Instead of subscribing to one method, I would like to argue for multiple strategies in teaching the history of medicine to students at health centers. I have not found any method to be a panacea and believe that an eclectic pragmatism ought to guide us at all times. Each approach to be selected must first take into consideration the particular institutional setting in which the teaching is going to be conducted. Numerous historical and political realities uniquely shape each academic environment thereby favoring or hindering specific prescriptions. Nowadays, few institutions retain a required course of medical history in their curriculum. If it exists as an elective, in what year is it offered? Is medical history considered to be part of the "basic" sciences or a handmaiden of clinical instruction? Does it share teaching time with other so-called "medical humanities" such as philosophy and literature? Even geography enters into the equation, since health centers are often separated from the rest of the university where historians may reside, or, as at Wisconsin, where the faculty of all basic sciences— including medical history—operates in facilities separated by almost a mile from clinicians.

Dr. Brieger claims to be a novice at this case-method approach, and if I interpret his remarks correctly, has invested five hours of the necessary 200 hours suggested as minimum preparation for the discussion of one single case. Therein lays one of the drawbacks of this procedure. Virtually all of the examples he proposes to present will require a great deal of research on the part of the instructor before they are sufficiently analyzed to merit the most elementary type of discussion with students.

Now let us assume that topics for case presentations are actually spin-offs of the teacher's current research interests, and may already have received enough scholarly scrutiny to be presented at a seminar. The problem then shifts to the students who may have difficulty coming up with their part of the equation, namely, completing a number of basic readings enabling them to participate and explore the issues. Without their sustained student input, the seminars will languish and turn into monologues by the instructor. In contrast, law students assiduously prepare for each case presentation, researching both the antecedents and context essential to a useful analysis. Similarly, medical house staff and faculty bone up for clinical case presentations, often reviewing pertinent literature, gathering statistical data, or analyzing previous case studies. These preparations, however modest and elementary in design, require a considerable amount of time, a commodity increasingly scarce in most crowded schedules at health centers. If the medical history course is organized in the midst of other time-consuming clinical rotations that often take students to distant hospitals and clinics, preparation time may be minimal and even attendance spotty: all factors militating against success.

Within the usual academic reward system that dictates students' priorities, clinical proficiency is already stressed over humanistic preparation, and this situation is partially responsible for decreased enrollments and participation in medico-historical activities. Paradoxically, this occurs more often when medical history is clearly identified as a separate discipline with specialized instructors and administrative independence. In fact, clinicians with historical avocations often have less trouble weaving their knowledge of the past into the day-to-day teaching, thus avoiding acrimonious turf disputes and the intense power play concerning slices of the curricular pie. Dubious claims about the utility of medical history notwithstanding, historians are seldom successful in such academic competitions.

Between 1971 and 1975, I conducted the issue-oriented seminar as an elective for freshmen medical students enrolled in our medical school. Student evaluations were positive but revealed the increasing competition for time with regular courses, and difficulties in completing reading assignments, term papers, and take-home examinations. After 1972, changes in the curriculum shifted a number of basic sciences from the second year back into the first, greatly overcrowding the latter. Moreover, medical history was at this time included in an expanding program of elective courses designed to aid students taking the required sequence. Thus, enrollments in the history of medicine elective, carrying only one academic credit, gradually dropped from a total of twenty-two students in 1971 to only six in 1975, while the total incoming class remained at 159 students.

With the addition of two new faculty members, our issue-oriented teaching was divided in 1976 into four distinct modules, each lasting four weeks. One seminar on women in medicine was taught by Judith Walzer Leavitt, stressing the sex of the patient as an important factor affecting nineteenth-century American medical practice. Another, presented by Ronald L. Numbers, examined the history of organized medicine in America and its effect on ethics, supply of medical physicians, cost of care, and the realities of medical power and politics. I myself gave two modules, one dealing with the history of the physician-patient relationship: its philosophical and religious underpinnings, the impact of the hospital, and technology as related to medical specialization. A final module examined the history of medical ethics, looking at the function of oaths, right to health, and medical malpractice and experimentation. Enrollment remained stationary with about eighteen students registering in 1976 and twelve in 1977.

In 1978, an issue-oriented reading course was only retained for our fourth-year medical students. Since most of the Wisconsin fourth-year curriculum in the medical school is composed of elective courses, students are able to select medical history for variable periods of time from an extensive catalogue of academic offerings. Since then, some have signed up with individual faculty members for variable periods of time from two to more than six weeks between clinical clerkships. This format allows time for in-depth reading and research no longer possible in the first year elective. Last year, for example, one student probed the origins of the family medicine movement in the United States and wrote a paper about his findings. Since he was going into a family residency program after graduation from medical school, this subject was of great interest to him.

At the same time, our department faculty decided to alter radically the format of the first-year elective for medical students and base instruction primarily on the use of films dealing with social, ethical, and institutional aspects of medicine. Beginning with an eight week program in 1978, we are now jointly offering sixteen presentations. Whenever possible, each film is introduced by one of the instructors with brief background statements to clarify both the context and to point out the main issues addressed in the film. Discussion following the film presentation is encouraged. Handouts containing lists of optional readings, topics for further discussion, and graphs or other materials are selectively provided to the class. Enrollment for the elective course rose dramatically over the last three years by about 120 students—and now includes approximately 75 percent of the entire incoming class.

I have personally tried to analyze the reasons for such a remarkable increase in student attendance. Not unexpectedly the evaluation forms convey a broad spectrum of reactions, ranging from the frivolous "I like movies" and "this is entertaining," to the more serious "I like to broaden my medical background," "gain a perspective," or simply "I am interested in history and the origins of medicine." These were among the most frequent responses to the question, "Why did you take this elective course?" reflecting a diversity of motivations and agendas that is probably representative of medical student populations elsewhere.

Indeed, the present generation of medical students, reared like their colleagues in other fields on a profusion of audio-visual stimuli—especially television—is of course highly receptive to instructional programs seeking to combine words and images. Student interest is frequently stimulated, lengthy explanations avoided, comprehension enhanced. Audio-visual aids have ceased to be the stepchildren of pedagogy, the last resort for an unprepared teacher to avoid embarrassment.

Moreover, looking at the individual rankings given to our presentations by the students, I feel that one of the principal reasons for the success of certain films in the classroom resides in their focus on human interest stories. The professional frustrations and personal tragedies of men like William Withering and Louis Pasteur depicted in films on the discovery of foxglove and the rise of bacteriology have been used by the media producers to illuminate the conceptual context and contemporary value-system, thereby pointing to issues and problems important in their time. The display of emotions and the revelation of eccentricities and foibles allow viewers to identify with the main protagonists of medical dramas played out against diverging historical backgrounds. The great men and women in medicine thus become life-size, instead of retaining an aura of superhuman perfection and dedication. In our recent experience, it is not uncommon to have medical students clap or boo during key scenes of certain films, reflecting an unexpected degree of involvement with the action.

These findings may be significant. Perhaps in our more recent quest to transcend purely anecdotal medical history, we may unwittingly have thrown out the baby with the bathwater. Our broad conceptual reconstructions of past healing can certainly be dry and impersonal abstractions. I can personally plead guilty for having stressed them. Maybe we need occasionally to add flesh and bones to our presentations, first linking past and present through perennial human situations before sketching the diverging attitudes and value-systems that characterized specific historical societies. I merely offer this as a suggestion for further experimentation in lectures, seminars, and especially audio-visual presentations.

A possible way of combining the advantages of case studies with in-depth reading and audio-visual supplements exists in health centers with independent study programs designed for students in their first two years of instruction. With federal support, our medical school initiated such a program of self-study in the early 1970s as an alternative to the official curriculum, and I was asked to develop a number of educational modules to be included as an elective. Specific learning objectives were systematically established for the students. The course utilized a number of readings, audio-cassettes, and films, explicitly listed among the activities for each module. Additional discussion periods with the faculty were built into the schedule to allow for students to emerge from their self-guided schooling and to be prepared to exchange impressions, voice criticisms, or demand advice. The elective status of the medical history course, and our eventual resolve to switch the entire first-year program to a simpler format based on films, ended for us this experience, but not before valuable feedback about the desirability of visual instructional materials was obtained. However, such an independent study plan could be a viable alternative at many institutions, especially those lacking specialized medical history faculty but able to purchase the necessary learning materials and provide other interested teachers for the discussions.

Before concluding, I would like to emphasize the importance of teaching medical history in a variety of postgraduate programs organized at health centers. Freed at last from the perennial race for grades, the constraints of an overloaded curriculum, and anxieties of acquiring minimal clinical skills, residents, fellows, and other recent medical graduates offer potential rewards to historians of medicine with pedagogical ambitions of modest scope. Rather than being comprehensive and systematic, teachers must learn to explain specific subjects and know how to link past and present concerns without distorting historical evidence and thereby jeopardizing their credibility.

Last year, for example, I organized on a weekly basis four informal seminars with residents from our Department of Family Medicine and Practice. Topics prepared for discussion were the history of concepts of health and sickness, medicine as a symbolic and cultural phenomenon, the role of medicine, and background of family medicine. Several faculty members joined the freewheeling exchanges, and our evaluations were quite encouraging. Another opportunity was the participation in grand rounds organized by the Department of Medicine. One topic was the clinical case history, an analysis of the changes that have occurred in the nature and gathering of clinical data. In another experiment, I attended for six months the weekly internal medicine staff conferences at the nearby Veterans Administration Hospital affiliated with our medical school. My presence allowed for considerable historical input concerning the ecology of illness, history of specific diseases, laboratory medicine, therapeutics, and other topics. This interaction frequently occurred either spontaneously at the time new admissions were presented by the house staff, or was carefully planned at least a week in advance to coincide with follow-up presentations of specific in-house cases.

Finally, the proliferation of postgraduate medical programs throughout the country also offers opportunities for teaching medical history. In Wisconsin, physicians have to complete fifteen hours of accredited continuing education per year to maintain their licenses to practice, and these conferences are increasingly in demand. In 1977, before the annual meeting of the American Association for the History of Medicine in Madison, both Chester Burns (University of Texas Medical Branch) and Robert Hudson (University of Kansas Medical Center) successfully conducted their day-long courses, sponsored by the Department of Continuing Medical Education in our Center for Health Sciences. Dr. Burns's seminar about the rights and duties in patient-physician relationships explored the Greek and Christian legacies, and ended with an examination of the Anglo-American experience before and after 1900. Dr. Hudson, in turn, organized his postgraduate seminar around the historical process of medical professionalization in America. Issues such as sectarianism, polypharmacy, education of physicians, and history of organized medicine were discussed in relation to past and present concerns. More than two thirds of the thirty-five persons enrolled in these programs were Wisconsin physicians, especially generalists and family practice oriented specialists. In their evaluation, they listed the discussion periods and newly acquired perspectives behind their daily efforts as highlights of the seminars.

These are just a few of the multiple opportunities awaiting medical historians in the teaching of medical history at health centers. Careful planning, intensive preparation including the use of audio-visual aids, and above all sensitivity to students' as well as physicians' needs and limitations can make these experiences both enjoyable and productive.

Notes

1. Guenter B. Risse, "W. S. Middleton and the Wisconsin chair in medical history: a unique tradition," *Bull. Hist. Med.*, 1976, *50:* 133–37.

2. I am grateful to Lloyd Stevenson for sharing with me Owsei Temkin's remarks made on 17 October 1979 following the showing of his videotape, and which will be published in the introduction to the volume commemorating the 50th anniversary of the Johns Hopkins Institute of the History of Medicine.

3. For a list and explanation of the topics see: Guenter B. Risse, "The role of medical history in the education of the 'humanist' physician: a re-evaluation," *J. Med. Ed.*, 1975, *59:* 465–68.

4. More details are contained in Guenter B. Risse, "Teaching medical history in the 1970s: new challenges and approaches," *Clio Medica*, 1975, *10:* 133–42.

MEDICAL HISTORY AND MEDICAL HUMANITIES: SOME NEW STYLES OF LEARNING AND TEACHING

Chester R. Burns

Patterns of learning and teaching in American medical schools labeled "medical humanities programs" have appeared only in the last dozen or so years. The first department of humanities in a medical school was established at the Pennsylvania State University School of Medicine at Hershey in 1967.[1] Data gathered for the American Medical Association's annual report on medical education for 1978–79 indicated that eighty-nine of 119 schools have established formal programs in the humanities, and seven others were planning such programs.[2] If administrators, faculty, and students are that serious about the "medical humanities," those interested in the future of medical history need to consider opportunities available in these new programs. Understanding these opportunities requires some historical perspective.

Gentleman Physicians

Only four years after receiving his medical degree from Edinburgh, Samuel Bard, in 1769, exhorted the medical graduates at King's College (now Columbia) to study the writings of Hippocrates and other physicians of antiquity. But, he said, "Do not affect the pedantry of despising the Moderns."[3] He urged them to study carefully the contributions of Sydenham, Boerhaave, Huxham, Pringle, and Whytt. The past of medicine (certainly its therapies) was vibrantly contemporary to Bard and his practitioner colleagues. Yet Bard pleaded for the medical moderns. Undergirding his rhetoric was a fundamental division between the knowledge of the ancients and that of modern thinkers who were rejecting or revising much of that classical learning, both medical and general.

Colleges and universities were institutions designed to transfer both "general" and "special" learning. But, how much general learning did a physician actually need? Did a knowledge of Greek and Latin make a discernible difference at the bedside of the sick? Answers to these two questions were rich with conflict for the slightly increasing number of American doctors who had had an opportunity to attend college before their medical studies. Most argued for as much general learning as possible. But most, echoing Benjamin Rush, had little use for Greek and Latin. Bloodletting and purging were the same whether recommended by Hippocrates or Boerhaave. Still, the number of doctors attending college gradually increased, and an eloquent minority believed that general, liberal studies were essential for "gentleman" physicians.

Doctors attended college because they wanted to be, and wanted to be viewed as "gentle" persons. The knowledge and skills acquired by liberal studies—so the ideal went—would automatically improve the general capabilities of any physician. These studies would prepare an individual for membership in a particular class of humans: the most extensively civilized one.

Humanities studies were the means to the ends of feeling superior, behaving civilly, and being judged as "gentle." Possession of a college degree meant possession of "higher" knowledge. Whether useful or not in treating the sick, this learning encouraged a physician to feel cultured. Classical languages and class privilege were intertwined, as were personal and professional respectability.

Those, including physician leaders, who cherished the humanities were facilitating the transfer of centuries of European culture and were also establishing and conserving the uniquely American values championed during the early decades of the new nation.

Before 1870, the senior-year course in moral philosophy was both symbol and bearer of these values. This course was a general study of human nature and included a mixture of history, religion, metaphysics, ethics, law, and perspectives from social sciences not yet separated from history and philosophy, such as psychology, economics, and political science.[5] Any student desiring a degree from most American colleges was expected to take this course. It was considered especially helpful for those entering the professions of law or ministry, but not medicine. Medical students were interested in natural philosophy and the natural sciences. John Gregory of Edinburgh and his Philadelphia disciple, Rush, even stipulated that studies in moral philosophy were inappropriate for those choosing medicine, hardly encouragement for any senior premed seeking connections between required college studies and professional aspirations, between knowledge of the humanities and medical skills.[6]

For most of the eighteenth and nineteenth centuries, this mattered little for the majority of practitioners because they had not studied in any American college. Apprenticeship was the primary path to the "special" knowledge needed by doctors. Caretakers of sick bodies learned what they needed to know by observation, imitation, and practice, not by reading passages in Greek and Latin, nor by taking courses in moral philosophy. After all, they wanted to be physicians, not preachers or lawyers. An eloquent few, though, wanted to be gentleman physicians.

Physicians as Scientists and Specialists

Between 1870 and 1930, a new set of professional ideals competed with the gentlemanly ones so dominant before that time. These values were more narrow, more pragmatic, and more democratic. They never completely replaced the imperatives of the old moral order, but, by 1930, they were becoming ascendant. Scientific knowledge and technical skills were essential features of this new set of values.

Acquiring scientific knowledge was more important than following any codified rule about respecting the allegedly superior learning of apprenticeship-trained, senior-citizen practitioners. During this time, thousands of American doctors went to Austria and Germany to learn the basic medical sciences of bacteriology, microbiology, and pathology, which were not being taught in their own schools.[7] Without that knowledge, they judged themselves inadequate as conscientious physicians. By 1930, the basic medical sciences were institutionalized in American medical schools, a process accompanied by a corresponding change in relationships between those schools and the American colleges educating future medical students.

Universities and medical schools had married for real; they were no longer related by name only. Premedical and medical studies were shaped into patterns of sequential learning: from physics, chemistry, and biology of high school and college to the anatomy, physiology, and biochemistry of medical school. To accomplish this, medical teachers engineered significant changes in premedical requirements: first, to four years of high school; then to one year of college; then, in 1918, to two years of college; and in 1953, to three years of college. The medical professors argued that these extensions permitted future physicians to master basic laboratory sciences, to become acquainted with the new behavioral and social sciences, and to receive some cultural polish from the old humanities. All this learning was expected to occur in the colleges, not in the medical schools.

Strikingly absent in the new marriage between the universities and the medical schools were sequences for the behavioral sciences, the social sciences, and the humanities, comparable to those of the physical and biological sciences. Professors in the medical schools seemed happy to leave the humanities and social sciences with the college teachers.[8]

By requiring more years of premedical study and by continually proclaiming the importance of a liberal education, medical educators believed that premeds would welcome their collegiate opportunities to become liberalized and humanized. Upon arriving at medical school, the premeds would possess cultural values and liberal skills; they would be "gentlemen." With their premedical studies in the natural sciences, these students would also be well prepared for the next developmental phases: becoming biomedical scientists and clinical specialists. Medical professors, unburdened of a need to teach cultural values, could concentrate on transmitting the scientific knowledge and developing the technical skills so essential to the new moral order of the medical profession.

Since the values attached to the old humanities were still, for most, grounded in the elitist ideals of the old gentlemanly schema, these dicta about premedical liberal studies unquestionably influenced a segment of physicians during this era. But three factors (at least) stimulated attitudes that ran counter to this particular style of marrying the two cultures for future physicians.

Democratization and social mobility affected medical education in profound ways. Photographs of medical school classrooms at the turn of the twentieth century depict hundreds of physician aspirants—with ties in place—eager to learn anatomy and biochemistry. The diploma mills and inferior schools of this time are well known. Although some of these students may have been charmed by the elitist norms of "gentleman" doctors, it is doubtful if most viewed class privilege and classical language as steps to personal and professional respectability. A "gentlemanly" attitude of moral superiority was not their forte.

A second factor encouraged resistance to the aristocratic model. The meaning of liberal education changed rapidly as an increasing number of American universities adopted an elective system of courses that gave prominent recognition to nonclassical and scientific studies. Those experiencing "higher education" no longer needed to take moral philosophy or know the classical languages; they could be liberalized with mathematics and biology. These changes were especially attractive to the new breed of premeds who were expected to confirm the importance of college studies as preparation for medical training, particularly the basic science part of that training.[9]

A third factor raised other doubts about the importance of the social sciences and humanities. This was the relative failure of most American physicians to participate in the transformation of the old moral philosophy into the social sciences and "scientific" humanities which took place between 1870 and 1930.[10] Few cared about the new organizations of professionals who constituted the Modern Language Association (1883), the American Historical Association (1884), the

American Economics Association (1885), the American Philosophical Association (1901), the American Political Science Association (1904), and the American Sociological Society (1905). Most physicians were far more concerned about scientific and technical developments in medicine proper, and were expressing those interests in new specialty societies emerging in the last quarter of the nineteenth century. They were as uninterested in the new social sciences as they had been in the old moral philosophy. They were obligated to care for sick bodies and their parts, not to tackle the economic, social, and political problems of the American culture. Burdensome enough were problems of wedding science to medical practice, of inventing new tools and mastering difficult techniques, of gaining social acceptance for the specialty organizations.

In becoming pathologists, internists, pediatricians, obstetricians, anesthesiologists, and surgeons, most doctors had no time for, or interest in, the social, historical, and philosophical sides of medicine. They could not become competent biomedical scientists and skilful clinical specialists, and also attend to the increasingly specialized domains of knowing being fashioned by a growing number of academic philosophers, economists, historians, sociologists, and political scientists.

However, when some of these social scientists and humanists began to study medicine as a major feature of American culture, some physician-educators began acknowledging the importance of these studies for future physicians. History and history of medicine were especially heralded as foci for integrating the old and the new, for correlating the humanities and the sciences.

Humanizing Physicians: Mostly History

As the twentieth century evolved, the size of the "dead" medical past increased as never before. William Osler knew nothing about insulin or cortisone. X-rays were never used on the patients of Samuel Gross. Harvey Cushing never prescribed penicillin. Halsted and Welch never observed the extraordinary developments in chest and heart surgery which occurred after 1940. Geriatrics, tranquillizers, organ transplantations—these were a few of the changes not even in the dreams of most nineteenth-century doctors. The results were twofold: a massive increase in the lode of medical ideas and practices no longer viable but of considerable interest to the historically minded, and an attitude among most scientists and clinicians that medicine's present and future were far more significant than its past.

Whenever the historically minded viewed that past, though, they perceived dedication, greatness, and progress. Historical studies could unite the best of cultural values with the best of professional ideals. Culture, science, and technology could be blended in future healers, who would carry forward the best of these traditions. As with history in the colleges, medical history in the medical schools became the preeminent humanities discipline.

The story of the teaching of medical history in the United States has been told in several studies, most recently by Genevieve Miller.[11] Only a few reminders are needed here. Sixty percent of the seventy-seven American medical schools offered regular courses in medical history by 1937. The need for historical understanding was so great that Johns Hopkins University established an academic unit in its medical school. Members of this unit would be expected to apply the school's cherished research model to the past of medicine. There would be full-time academic researchers and teachers in medical history. These professionals would be able to apply the best research methods in conducting their studies, and they would be equipped to respond to those who felt they needed the historical understanding for their humanization.

The new group of professional medical historians was faced with two rather awesome challenges: developing a comprehensive and detailed view of past human experiences with health and disease, using the most refined techniques of "scientific" historiography; and creating strategies that would allow those views of the past to prevent future physicians from becoming dehumanized by their scientific and technical training, or, at best, to nurture the biomedical sciences and clinical specialists into loving, caring healers. Both challenges constituted an enormous and unrealistic burden. But several of the professional historians, such as Sigerist, Shryock, and Rosen, gallantly responded to these expectations.

Henry Sigerist, who became director of the Institute of the History of Medicine at Johns Hopkins in 1932, was the first full-time professionally trained historian of medicine in the United States who championed all of the perspectives of the critical approach to medico-historical scholarship. He was neither hobbyist nor antiquarian; he was committed to rigorous historical investigation "for its own sake." Sigerist was also an "applied" historian, using and teaching history as part of the quest for more effective health care delivery systems. Richard Shryock, focusing on the Anglo-American experience, wedded the riches of social and cultural history to the central features of medical science and practice, and unhesitatingly depicted and interpreted the recent past and its bearings on the present. George Rosen continuously searched for relationships between the medical past and its present and future, especially as those relationships affected policy decisions in public-health practices. Rosen theorized, because he believed in a rational foundation for health care delivery; he joined together history and sociology in order to lay that foundation. Sigerist, Shryock, and Rosen all hoped that their historical studies would make a practical difference in the level of self-understanding among physicians and health care professionals, in the care of the sick and the healthy, and in the creation of more adequate public policies for dealing with the myriad problems of providing suitable health care.[12]

Rewarding differences must have occurred for many students and practitioners alike. Medical history was supported as never before, with books, journals, societies, courses. In 1955, one survey indicated that 88 percent of medical schools in the United States were offering elective or required courses. By 1970, twelve medical schools had departments or divisions and six offered graduate degrees in medical history. History of medicine had been established as a specialty in some academic health centers. For those who believed in scholarship "for its own sake," a future seemed assured.[13]

Historical studies could represent "objective," "detached," and "uninvolved" inquiry into events of the medical past, with accurate stories as the predictable outcomes. The value of this research model of medical history can hardly be questioned by those whose concern is with truth and accuracy, fact over fiction. But the events of professionalization in medical history brought about by the dedicated theoreticians and practitioners of "critical" history created frustrations for those who wanted history to be *the* institutionalized tactic for humanizing physicians.

Scientists, clinicians, and educators could not perceive the humanizing effects of medico-historical studies, nor could they, upon reflection, really expect historical methods alone to accomplish these objectives. History became for them a focus on the dead part of human existence; it was a posture of escapism and denial, reinforced by historians writing only for other historians. Historical studies were coldly analytical and absurdly comprehensive, not appropriate for the education of empathetically caring and realistically specialized doctors. Progressive history of medicine fueled the paternalistic and self-righteous tendencies of a medical profession already being called upon to respond more adequately to the cries of anguished citizen-patients and the demands of fellow health care professionals who wanted equal status. While students were clamoring for involvement and breadth, professional historians were becoming more detached and narrow.[14] Earlier enthusiasms for medical history as a humanizing strategy waned as the second half of the twentieth century evolved. Taking its place were interests in other humanities and social disciplines.

Humanizing Physicians: Plus or Minus History?

In 1965, two years before the first department of humanities was established in an American medical school, the United States Congress created the National Endowment for the Humanities as a Federal agency that would provide grants in support of research and education in the humanities. The following fields are included in the NEH circumscription of the humanities: history, philosophy, languages, literature, linguistics, archaeology, jurisprudence, history and criticism of the arts, ethics, comparative religion, and those aspects of the social sciences employing historical or philosophical approaches. Excepting history, these fields were not institutionalized significantly in medical schools before the late 1960s.

Since that time, their institutionalization has occurred steadily, but not without conflict and stress. During a time of enormous technical changes in medical practices, with their accompanying value conflicts, programs in ethics and philosophy have received new vitality.[15] On the other hand, literature and languages have received scant attention. No more than ten programs (probably less) have been systematic, intentional efforts to nurture and support teachers representing two or more humanities fields.[16] Only a few historians have worked in these programs.

As one of them, I acknowledge some trepidation about offering any generalizations. Humanities education in American academic health science centers is still in a neonatal phase. Nevertheless, a few observations may encourage some historians to participate more actively in these new endeavors.

Not a few of the new humanities teachers in health care professional schools appear to ignore the story of the teaching of medical history in American medical schools. Such inattention and ignorance may follow from a desire to avoid some of the unrealistic expectations associated with past historical teaching. Sadly, though, such condescension has allowed too many philosophers and ethicists, for example, to exhibit another set of unrealistic expectations about the roles of humanists in academic health centers. The logical and definitional nuances of the ethicists are viewed by the students as esoteric and nonsensical abstractions, just as the students dismiss the memory treadmills proffered by some history teachers. The philosophers' word-webs add confusion, not clarity. Those who suffer the most from their arrogances are the students, the future practitioners.

But not for long. In responding to the expectations generated by the values of scientific knowledge and technical expertise, the students cull the irrelevancies with racetrack speed. They embrace the opposite with a similar intensity, which helps to explain their fervent support of medical humanities studies that respond to their needs, both vocational and personal. Students and their needs are the primary reason for the rapid development of medical humanities courses and programs since 1967. Today's students are not satisfied with science and technology alone, but they also reject humanists and social scientists who model only a technical expertise in their discipline, who cannot translate from the laboratory (or library) to the real world of health care practice for today and tomorrow.

I am not condemning the technical expertise, the scholarship "for its own sake." It is absolutely necessary and I categorically reject the dilettantes who pretend they are qualified to teach in academic health centers, whatever their subject area. But the scholarly preparation symbolized by a Ph.D. is not sufficient. Humanities scholars and social scientists must learn how to use their knowledge and their investigative approaches in ways that meet the needs of future health care practitioners. This is the second of the awesome challenges mentioned before: How to apply humanities and social science disciplines most effectively in the education of future healers!

If historians and others genuinely want to be integral components of academic health centers, they must not ignore this second challenge. They must learn how to enrich the memory banks of every student; how to respond to the defensive fears of nonhistorian colleagues who, denying the value of understanding traditions, repeat past mistakes; how to achieve some pedagogical versatility in the broad and varied continuum of health professional education; how to win support for exploring new patterns of historical teaching in humanities and social sciences contexts.[17]

These contexts do not provide panaceas. They do provide a construct of institutional and conceptual realities that may be more realistic and stable than any heretofore attempted. They may provide a base for actually testing the persistent hypothesis that humanities studies are causally significant in the creation of civil and gentle healers.

Notes

1. Sam A. Banks, "The newcomers: humanities and social sciences in medical education," *Tex. Rep. Biol. Med.,* 1974, *32:* 19–30.

2. "Medical education in the United States, 1978–79," *J.A.M.A.,* 7 March 1980, *243:* 857–58.

3. Samuel Bard, *A Discourse upon the Duties of a Physician* (New York: A. & J. Robertson, 1769), p. 7

4. Kevin P. Bunnell, "Liberal education and American medicine," *J. Med. Educ.,* 1958, *33:* 319–40.

5. Wilson Smith, *Professors and Public Ethics Studies of Northern Moral Philosophers Before the Civil War* (Ithaca, N.Y.: Cornell University Press, 1956); see especially chapter 2.

6. Chester R. Burns, "American medical ethics: some historical roots," in *Philosophical Medical Ethics: Its Nature and Significance,* ed. S. F. Spicker and H. T. Engelhardt, Jr. (Dordrecht, Holland: D. Reidel, 1977), pp. 21–26.

7. Thomas Bonner, *American Doctors and German Universities* (Lincoln: University of Nebraska Press, 1963).

8. Since most of these teachers knew little about the biomedical sciences, they could not have been expected to demonstrate the relevance of their humanities or social sciences discipline to medicine.

9. The hegemony of science studies in molding the myth of the premed is still a basic feature of college education today. But changes are occurring. See John T. Bruer and Kenneth S. Warren, "Liberal arts and premedical curriculum," *J.A.M.A.*, 23/30 January 1981, *245:* 364–66.

10. Most of the physicians who did participate in this transformation were members of the American Academy of Medicine. This organization will be described in a separate study.

11. Genevieve Miller, "Medical history," in *The Education of American Physicians: Historical Essays,* ed. Ronald Numbers (Berkeley: University of California Press, 1980), pp. 290–308.

12. Numerous writings confirm these generalizations; see the following bibliographies: Genevieve Miller, ed., *A Bibliography of the Writings of Henry E. Sigerist* (Montreal: McGill University Press, 1966); idem, "Bibliography of Richard H. Shryock," *J. Hist. Med.,* 1968, *23:* 8–15; idem, "George Rosen: bibliography," in *Healing and History,* ed. Charles E. Rosenberg (New York: Science History Publications, 1979), pp. 252–62.

13. Chester R. Burns, "History in medical education: the development of current trends in the United States," *Bull. N.Y. Acad. Med.,* 1975, *51:* 862–63.

14. Dramatically exemplifying some of these tensions are two book reviews published in *Bull. Hist. of Med.,* 1980, *55:* 131–40.

15. Chester R. Burns, "Medical ethics and jurisprudence," in Numbers, *Education of American Physicians,* pp. 273–89.

16. For a survey of sixty-five medical humanities programs, see Thomas K. McElhinney, ed., *Human Values Teaching Programs for Health Professionals* (Ardmore, Pa.: Whitmore Publishing Co., 1981).

17. I have offered some practical suggestions in the paper cited in n. 13 and in the following: "Exploring new possibilities in the teaching of medical history," *Clio Medica,* 1975, *10:* 143–52 and "Liberating medical minds: can history help?," in *The Role of the Humanities in Medical Education,* ed. Donnie J. Self (Norfolk, Va.: Bio-Medical Ethics Program, 1978), pp. 8–20. An excellent introduction to the humanities as they bear on contemporary medical education is the group of essays by Edmund Pellegrino collected under the title *Humanism and the Physician* (Knoxville: University of Tennessee Press, 1979).

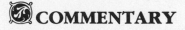COMMENTARY

Todd L. Savitt

Dr. Burns has very neatly and clearly provided us with a historical perspective on the teaching of humanities and history in medical schools. From his presentation we can better understand the derivation of our roles in medical education today. I would like now to look closer at the present scene in medical history and medical humanities and propose new roles and new directions for our historical endeavors.

Dr. Burns explained how medical education lost its link with the traditional humanities and turned to the natural, medical, and now even behavioral sciences. Medical history as a discipline, imported from Europe and planted in American medical schools, has not always taken root, flourished, and spread. Too many recipients of our teaching have not picked our flowers or taken our cuttings to plant in their own gardens. We have become isolated from the present concerns of medicine. We hide behind elitist, specialized studies of the past.

This characterization is, of course, not true of all medical historians, but does accurately reflect a trend. We have too often chosen to ignore current issues in favor of "pure" history. As Dr. Burns and others have shown in their writings, medical history in medical schools has lost popularity and curriculum time. Can this negative attitude and trend be reversed?

The program with which I have been involved for the past five years has opened my eyes to new possibilities. Medical humanities—in not exactly the classical form Dr. Burns described—offers historians a route back into the mainstream of medical education. Human values programs, to use the current catch-phrase (and I exclude here those programs which are really directed toward the "completion of being" or toward straight behavioral sciences), can draw historians out of isolation without diluting or contaminating the discipline. Too few of us are familiar with the Society for Health and Human Values or the *Hastings Center Reports*. Too few of us have talked seriously with philosophers of medicine, medical ethicists, medical anthropologists, sociologists, economists, and those interested in literature and medicine, in order to work out ways of bringing future physicians' attention to the medical nonsciences. Medical humanities is a way for us historians to introduce our discipline to students, and to gain some unexpected side benefits. Instead of fighting with ethicists, behavioral scientists, and economists for a slice of the medical curricular pie, we can join with these people in designing integrated, broad-spectrum, "interdisciplinary," introductory courses. All medical humanities program faculty would co-teach such courses and would also then teach spin-off, disciplinary courses offered to the now more knowledgeable, more mature, more thoughtful junior and senior medical students (and even residents). Medical students could be offered courses such as "Social and Ethical Issues in Medical Practice" early in their careers. These classes would provide a general perspective of the medical world, and introduce them to the wide variety of issues facing medicine and the wide variety of disciplines from which those issues can be discussed. Later in their careers students could choose either to look more deeply into one of those disciplines and learn *its* perspective on the medical world, or to think broadly again by choosing another integrated course. These integrated courses, by the way, need to be academically strict but also vital, not watered down lecture courses with no content or serious requirements. Students should be graded and expected to think, discuss, and write. Some students will complain, but most will accept, enjoy, and learn.

At risk of becoming too personal or sounding arrogant about a moderately successful program, I will describe the arrangement at the University of Florida, not only because it is the one with which I am most familiar, but also because I believe it is reproducible. (Of course each school has its own unique financial and organizational situation, but the basic idea of a medical humanities program presented here can be adapted to meet those variations.) Five of us comprise a Division of Social Sciences and Humanities within the Department of Community Health and Family Medicine. The disciplines represented are medical history, medical sociology and public policy, medical anthropology, philosophy of medicine, and medical ethics/theology. Each of us has a joint appointment with our disciplinary department on campus. Other programs around the country have different combinations: for instance, Galveston's faculty includes people in law and American studies as well as history and ethics; Hershey's has teachers of medical literature, art, and photography in addition to philosophy and, until very recently, history. Stony Brook and Southern Illinois University have other variations in their medical humanities programs.

Our Division of Social Sciences and Humanities at the University of Florida has formal contact with the medical students throughout their four years. Incoming first-year students learn about our existence during orientation week when they participate, in classes of twenty, in two required Ethics Case Conferences led by a member of the Division and a clinician. Part of their introduction to anatomy and cadavers at the end of orientation week includes Savitt's slide and film presentation on the history of anatomical study, "Resurrection and Dissection." About fifteen to twenty students come regularly to monthly brown-bag noon-hour history of medicine talks throughout the year. For seven weeks, shortly before these students begin their clinical clerkships in the latter part of the second year, the Division of Social Sciences and Humanities teaches a required course called "Social and Ethical Issues in Medical Practice." We divide up the class of 120 into groups of about twenty and discuss various topics facing modern medicine in fourteen, two hour sessions. Required readings range over all our disciplines, as do the discussions. Each of us, of course, adds his or her own emphases and perspectives in the classroom. We also require every student to write short, weekly reflection papers and a longer term paper: all to encourage them to reason through, in an informed way, their own thoughts on a particular topic or reading. Then, during the clerkship year, each of us works with students in one way or another. I spend one day every two weeks observing and discussing students' interaction with patients in the examining rooms of one of the department's rural health clinics. This is a fine way regularly to keep the realities of health and sickness and of doctor/patient relationships before me as I do my historical research, writing, and teaching. It is, in many ways, the highlight of my work at the University of Florida. During the students' fourth year, about eight to ten choose to take a history of medicine elective where we trace in some depth the development of modern medicine and also hit upon the students' particular interests. These classes, because of their size, lend themselves to discussions of past and present issues.

Our division is represented on the orientation and curriculum committees of the medical school, so that we have direct input into the planning of the University of Florida's medical education program. Because we view medical education as a continuum which begins in the undergraduate years and extends through and beyond residency work, we offer courses at each of these levels. Throughout a University of Florida student's program he or she inevitably bumps into medical humanities and, more especially for our purposes here, medical history.

We historians should be prepared, in teaching medical humanities courses, to sacrifice a bit of depth (and here is the sticky part) to get students thinking about the profession they are entering. Historians have been loathe to "spot teach." Medical history, we too often assert, requires a knowledge of events and ideas from ancient primitives to the germ theory and beyond. I believe we can compromise a bit on this. Medical history is appealing enough that we will always attract some students to go further and gain more historical depth. But it is hopeless to force feed an entire medical class. (I have discovered that I have been too timid in introducing medical history into my humanities classes.

They usually ask for more.) I don't think there is danger of losing
students or of seriously distorting the ideas and materials presented.

Integrated and cooperative courses can do wonders for both
students and teachers. Faculty development is well served by inter-
disciplinarity. Instead of working solely with other historians or with
clinicians, why not work also with philosophers, theologians, and social
scientists? We then share offices, face common problems, read each
other's papers, discuss issues from our different perspectives, and
broaden *our* worlds. These new ideas then get transmitted to our
students. We do not cease being historians simply because we teach
humanities. On the contrary, we learn from our new colleagues. We
may find the differences in thinking and approach of some of our new
nonhistorian colleagues unacceptable or not understandable. The
"mind set" of the social scientist, for example, may seem terribly,
almost treasonously different from our own. But one can deal with this
and learn from it.

Clinical faculty development and improved understanding between
clinical and humanities faculty members are other benefits of such a
program. On my way up here to Baltimore, a clinician colleague and I
were talking in the Atlanta airport. As a regular participant in our
undergraduate courses he had read William Carlos Williams's short
story, "The Girl with a Pimply Face," as had the third-year medical student he was working with this week at one of our department's rural
health clinics. In discussing one particular patient about whom both felt
a little uneasy, the clinician compared the girl they had just seen to the
girl in the story. Both instantly understood the young patient's situation
and each other. Though this incident is not an example from history, it
does point out how our involvement in medical humanities can aid the
teaching and practice of medicine.

Before concluding, I would like to interject one caveat. Words like
humanities, humanism, and human values are much used in medical cir-
cles today, often without any real understanding. Too frequently, what
goes on in medical schools under the rubric of humanities or human
values in medicine is either really (a) a disguised social/behavioral
science program where emphasis is placed on self-fulfillment, or (b) a
strictly medical-ethics program without classical humanities components like philosophy and history. It seems to me that humanities and
medicine programs need to include, at a minimum, history and ethics/
philosophy. Courses in these disciplines necessarily and almost
automatically raise questions of human values which can be discussed
in the modern context. As I said earlier, we should go so far as to integrate history with other disciplines in the humanities and let students
see how the past ties in with present-day concerns.

As must be evident, even after almost five years in the Florida program I am still enthusiastic and committed to the humanities approach, for both my own and my students' sakes. Not every activity I am involved in at the University of Florida's medical school is directly or even remotely related to history. But my historian's mind is always working, drawing historical material or concepts together whenever appropriate in the classroom or clinic. Students know me as a historian first, but also as one interested in concerns ranging from rural health practices to the state of medical education today and in the past. I feel that I am a better teacher for having been forced to look at both the past and present in medicine. We historians do not, of course, by becoming involved in medical humanities courses, become experts in medical literature, medical ethics, or health policy. But we can help students think through their own ideas and opinions on a variety of topics. We can even provide them with sources and a historical view of the questions they pose. Medical history does teach human values just as philosophy, ethics, and literature do. The Society for Health and Human Values needs historians to broaden its vision. It is lonely now at those meetings. Ethics dominates the discussions. We can also become so deeply involved in the curricular workings of our medical schools that our presence would be missed. Without losing our professional identities we historians of medicine can and should work more closely with other humanities disciplines to better ourselves, our chosen profession, and our future physicians.

DISCIPLINARY PERSPECTIVES IN THE HISTORY OF MEDICINE: A VIEW FROM THE 1980s

Russell C. Maulitz

Try as I might, I find it hard to evade the feeling that somewhere the man who was born just over a century ago, the man who was known as the Sage of Baltimore, Popsy's old friend and sparring partner H. L. Mencken, is watching these proceedings and smiling rather broadly. Perhaps not so broadly that the cigar would fall from the side of his mouth, but enough to indicate his smug satisfaction at knowing what to expect when those who teach something get together to talk about teaching it.

Mr. Mencken really did not hold truck with those who made it their business to talk about pedagogy. He thought it best, presumably, just to get on with the job, however that might be defined. If we take heed of this today, are we stymied from the start? Not necessarily, if we recognize that today's is—or should be—a signal occasion for finding better ways to get on with our job; that is, to reanimate the history of medicine as it is practiced in our health professional schools. It is fitting that we make the effort.

I want to try to contribute in a small way to this effort; but I also want to avoid bringing down the ethereal wrath of old H. L. by pretending to have new pedagogical answers, and talking about how I teach. I would therefore like to be indulged in a certain old-fashioned conceit. That conceit is simply that there really is an organic relationship, a symbiosis of some sort, between our research and our teaching in medical history. Hardly a startling assertion. Many have made it before. No doubt there are shearing forces that separate our research and teaching interests, especially when it comes to teaching in the medical curriculum.[1] But I will proceed as though what is worth *investigating* in the medical center is worth *teaching* there. What this means on the ground may be no more than the observation that people teach an audience best when the subject is exciting to them as well.

Let us assume, then, that there is indeed a nexus of interest representing and uniting the loosely bounded discipline of medical history, tying together investigation and education into an axial, disciplinary core. Where has this interest been in the past, where is it now, and where is it going in the next decade? The last part of the question is perhaps the most arresting, since the answer (or answers) to it will have a great deal of influence on our audiences and resources in the years ahead. Can we expect the medical schools to maintain a sustaining level of proprietary concern about the care and feeding of medical history? Or has its core of interest shifted so far away from the preoccupations of the health science centers that now, untethered by shared meaning, it threatens to collapse into other areas of significance and concern?

If we are to plot a course for the future, it seems appropriate first to turn our analytical tools on our own past progress.[2] We can look at the utilities that medical history has previously been perceived to offer, and also glance at its patrons and its disciplinary near-neighbors in medical education. If we do so, we begin to see that our discipline, like many of the objects of its study, has its own several pasts and its own possible futures. We can begin to see it, that is, within its medical context as an emerging discipline that was characterized, as it evolved, by certain historically defined relations between patrons and practitioners, and by certain external boundaries, historically defined by the disciplinary neighbors ringing it.

What *did* a sense of the past mean to our counterparts and their patrons in earlier periods? Lord Acton once said that "the man who is not consciously aware of the Past as his own history has no character," and the medical school supporters of this dictum seem, over the years, to have concurred. History builds strong character twelve ways. But the quality and nature of that character have, like the chameleon, changed along with the sense of the *utility* of the medical history.

There was a time when medicine and its history were virtually coextensive. Many have made that point before in public forums of this sort. For the longest time—essentially down to the nineteenth century—medical history was medical doctrine because it represented medical authority. History represented such authority with an immediacy that is apparent even in the work of those figures—from the Renaissance through the Scientific Revolution of the seventeenth and eighteenth centuries—whom we recognize as innovators.

Even in the early nineteenth century, the sense of historical distance was small intellectually; hence there was little or no social gap between physician and historian. More often than not, they were one and the same. The utility of history was direct, clinical, practical—and conservative. Under the banner of Hippocratism, for example, most physicians perceived authority in their historical discourse as congruent with that in their other disciplines. When the boundaries were thus indistinct, there could be little talk of "disciplinary neighbors"; it was a matter of "every physician his own historian." It is likely that patronage was not an issue under such a regime.

This picture began to undergo a sea-change sometime in the early decades of the nineteenth century. As the idea and ideologies of science and professionalism began in tandem to make inroads into medicine, transforming its face irrevocably, the value of history to its practitioners was itself changed, pushed back to a status at the same time more distanced and more immanent.[3] Medical history was no longer merely the repository of scientific authority, but rather the legitimator of medical men's changing aspirations. As the new science and the new professional sense of identity became cognitively distanced from the old wisdom, the sense of a hallowed and far-reaching past took on a different cultural utility.

This new utility had two aspects. On the one hand, clinical elites from Laennec to Osler could see the value of fostering medical history in terms of rituals of acculturation. Professional mentalities required the sanctification of history as the professional role emerged from its baser craft and proprietary roots. On the other hand, the new Brahmins of scientific medicine from Billroth to Welch were similarly concerned, as the nineteenth century wore on, to encapsulize and sanctify the paths they had followed to the new scientific ethos. Their new scientific credo required not historical authority, but a historical rationale, a valuation to be placed on the *slope* of the cognitive growth curve.[4]

The transition from history as authoritative and immediate to history as legitimizing and immanent represented the crossing of a Great Divide in the development of the discipline. On this, the near side of the Great Divide, the role of the historian crystallized out in a flesh-and-blood creature, responsible for a circumscribed body of knowledge. He was now responsible *to* certain people as well: at times to his neighbors in the new entrepreneurial, biomedical disciplines; and at times to his patrons among the clinical elite. This responsibility did not foreclose his attempting to instill a sense of conscience along with a transcendent sense of legitimacy. It did mean, however, that his central approach to history would remain what George Rosen has labeled "iatrocentric."[5] Virchow may have been the theorist of the cell-state as well as of the cell, but the historians focused only on his life and theory, not on the cellular individual—not on the patient or the lower orders of practitioners.

If this new mentality was evident by the late nineteenth century, when exactly had it supervened? When did medical history cross that first Great Divide? It is only a small evasion to point out that shifts in mentalities usually occur over bands of time rather than at fixed points. Along the way, however, there usually are indicators of these shifts, perhaps in the form of publishing milestones. Thus we might look at the critical four decades between 1840 and 1880 and cite two specific indicators of the shift I have been discussing. Sigerist, for one, pointed out this transition in terms of the imputed value of the classical sources. He noted in his essay "On Hippocrates" that the great European editions of the ancients in modern translation were avowedly intended for different audiences. When Littré published the first volume of his Hippocratic canon in 1839, he stated his conviction that it was still useful for medical practitioners. In 1861, the tenth volume appeared. Littré noted that it was published primarily for the use of the medical historian.[6]

A publishing event at the very end of the mid-nineteenth-century decades of transition exemplified in an equally elegant manner the shift in attitudes toward medical knowledge, and hence medical history. I am thinking actually of a closely timed *pair* of events in 1879 and 1880, namely, the publication of the first volumes, respectively, of the *Index Medicus* and the *Index-Catalogue.*[7] Though the *Index-Catalogue* was begun first, the *Index Medicus,* which fulfilled more immediate needs, was published first. As a guide to the holdings of the library of the Surgeon General's Office, the *Index-Catalogue* was intended to have hermeneutic value as well as serve as a mere compilation. It could be seen as a roadmap for the growing discipline of medical history. Recognizing the importance of meeting the need for access to current information, John Shaw Billings and his patrons could have neglected the historic overview of medicine offered by the contents of the *Index-Catalogue;* they could just have produced the *Index Medicus* by itself, or collapsed the *Index Catalogue* into it. Instead, they gave history what they felt was its due, which happened to be equivalent to (if not greater than) the supposed importance of current medical informational needs. In the field of medicine in America in the 1880s, as in its European counterpart of the preceding decades, history enjoyed a newly distanced, but still immanent value. In 1880, the double face of Janus was an image that had concrete meaning for the American man of medicine.[8]

Beginning at this time, somewhere between 1880 and 1910, another fissure within medicine—another Great Divide—began to grow wider. Now even the elite of medicine began to splinter. Fault lines deepened between those whose interests revolved around patient care, and those whose concerns revolved around research in the laboratory.[9] These cleavages within the elites of medicine were mapped onto the output of medical historians. Their resulting work became then (as it is sometimes now) not only celebrations of the past but implicit programmatic statements about the current agendas of medicine. The classic example of such a text is Knud Faber's *Nosography,* which brilliantly described the work of the clinical greats of the late nineteenth century, even as it sought to ensure a place in the sun for their twentieth-century progeny.[10]

Even with these cleavages, however, the received wisdom of late nineteenth-century iconology survived intact well into our own century. The compacting and bounding-off of medical history by the end of the nineteenth century did not lead initially to its decimation in the schools of medicine, but rather to a new triumphalism, a further shoring-up of the aspirations of the institution builders of the last century. This triumphalism was responsible for much of the self-exemplifying institution building in the history of medicine (and incidentally, in the history of science) that occurred in the first half of this century.[11]

What has happened since then? Who are the inheritors? In terms of patrons and potential audiences, the sense of distance from the past—both social and cognitive—has undergone yet another sea-change. This final shift began not with Viet Nam, although widespread disenchantment with professional elites may have accelerated the process at that time, but with the rise of state-funded "big medicine" in the interwar and (especially) post–World War II periods. I ascribe the change to a concomitant shift in the essential character of the patrons of medical history, and, in fact, the character of most of the leaders of medical education in general. The entrepreneurial elite who enacted the changes responsible for the heady atmosphere and institutional experimentation of the Flexner era has given way to a managerial/technocratic elite responsible for the care and feeding of normal science and standard practice. The result, a pious triumphalism of future promise, is a form of *hubris* that, ironically, accords with a central tenet of medicine's bitterest critics: the abandonment of the triumphalism of the past. The twin religion of science and professionalism, now the established faith, can afford to dispense with a past that seems increasingly remote and otiose. Medical history, no longer needed to lend legitimacy to the entrepreneurs who participated in ringing its changes, ceases to play even a residual, immanent role.

A word, finally, about the most recent patrons and audiences of medical history—admittedly in the main outside the conventional medical schools—namely, those connected with the stream often lumped (somewhat unjustly) under the rubric of revisionist history. The old iatrocentric history is finding its nemesis in a new spirit of what one might call iatroclasm—iatroclastic history—stressing medicine as it has been historically practiced on the ground and experienced by the patient.[12] A new skepticism about the healing role replaces the stale triumphalism of earlier periods. The hue and cry that results when the problem of explaining *innovation* and the individual actor's contribution is brought up, however, raises what is probably a sham issue. Individual figures may be given their due by the historian who recognizes them as actors interacting with a variety of larger contexts. When the dust from the fallen idol settles, I think we will be able to see past the traces of the giants to the habitat beyond, and I am optimistic about the lessons to be learned from it. I think we may be surprised at how receptive some of the new managers of health education may be, if we can begin to yoke this and other recent currents of historical interest into a few coherent conceptual streams.

It seems to me that we are on the verge of something like this process of intellectual synthesis. Where will the process take us? And what sort of interface will remain with the medical center as we take the next step? My crystal ball is as murky as the next fellow's, but I think it takes no great prescience to see medical history moving forward along at least three broad disciplinary fronts. For want of better terms, I will call these fronts contemporary history, global history, and interpretive history. Each of these three fronts represents a borderland between the discipline and new neighbors, or at least a newly widened border with old neighbors. As to the prospects of finding utility, and hence patrons, within the health professional schools, let me say at the outset that I consider those prospects surprisingly good, for the oldest and perhaps best of reasons: mutual self-interest.

Allow me to elaborate. The first borderland I see the discipline exploring is that shared with the contemporary historian, the public historian, and the policy analyst. Historically, there seems to be a felt need, as each century draws towards a close, to begin to delineate the history of medicine in that century. Hence we are beginning now to see what our predecessors saw one hundred years ago: the writing of the history of science and medicine in our own century. But "as the historian of medicine approaches nearer to his own times, he finds his path encumbered with almost insurmountable difficulties. The subject on which he has to tread differs, perhaps, from every other branch of science in this circumstance, that our actual information does not increase . . . in proportion to our experience." [13] The last two sentences were first written not in 1980, but almost a century and a half before by the English physician-historian, John Bostock.

Bostock was not the last observer to express anxiety about doing the history of contemporary and near-contemporary medicine. This uneasiness, which many of us may share, is itself rather interesting and deserving of historical scrutiny. On rereading Bostock, we find that his concerns grow more complex. At first glance, the first part of Bostock's statement, in which he voices his plaint over the "path encumbered," resonates with our own difficulties in coping with the welter of scientific information and clinical developments comprising twentieth-century medicine. We take a gander at the luxuriant growth of underbrush that has overgrown the path of medicine over the past seventy-five years, whet the blades of our historical machete knives, and start hacking away.

But when Bostock complained in 1835 that "our . . . information does not increase in proportion to our experience," he wasn't, as we discover on repeated reading, referring to an information explosion. He was talking about an *experiential* explosion with which the then rapidly evolving sciences—including those, such as chemistry and physiology, thought to be closely linked with medicine—simply couldn't keep up. The weight of this argument seems to rest on two struts. First, Bostock was saying, experience remained a central source of learning, irreplaceable by theoretical sciences, both because of the necessity for mastering clinical technique and because of the ethical limitations on the use of experimental science at the bedside. I think he was also saying, secondly and somewhat paradoxically, that clinical regimes—unlike scientific dicta—have a finite half life. The "narrator" of recent change—Bostock's contemporary historian—gave a "favourable report [of it], yet in the space of a few short years the boasted remedy has lost its virtue." [14]

Perhaps the situation described by Bostock, as he faced the very real problems of looking back and describing the changes he had witnessed over the first third of the nineteenth century, isn't so different from the one we face today. Perhaps it is the tension we feel, between the explosiveness and the emphemerality of knowledge, that is in fact the hallmark of the historian of contemporary medicine. Both qualities are now felt most poignantly in our health professional schools. For the medical schools, I think it will become a matter of obligation and equity—particularly on the North American continent, which first occupied the center of the world medical stage in the twentieth century—to support this part of the new medical history.

The second genre representing the new terrain toward which I believe medical history will inevitably expand is what I have called global history. In the work of people as diverse as William McNeill, Rosemary Stevens, and Matthew Ramsay we have already seen our near-neighbors in the history of education, epidemiology, policy analysis, European social history, and a number of other areas beginning to use the tools of comparative history to tackle some of the most refractory problems in current historiography. A number of the problems that our health professional schools have only recently been forced to confront seems uniquely susceptible to this sort of historical analysis. I am thinking in particular of issues like the fate of the hierarchy of health professions, the problem of equity in the distribution of health services, and the nature of the doctor-patient (or as it is now fashionably called, the client-provider) relationship. Each of these issues has historically been approached in a variety of ways in different national cultures. As yet there are precious few examples of this sort of work, but a few hardy souls have begun to venture seriously into cross-cultural history.[15]

Historians have just begun to demonstrate how these health practices have diverged in a context-dependent manner, both within Western medical cultures and between Western and non-Western traditions. In the late twentieth century the importance of this process of divergence, and the possibility of future convergence, has taken on a new immediacy. There are some specific reasons for this. One is that, while it has become a cliché to note the increasing interdependence of national cultures and contexts, it is also a fact. Another corollary reason is the increasing importance of the Third World. The significance of such developments goes beyond polishing the image and the judgment of our policy makers, health oriented or not, in government and in the international relations network. Increasingly the interdependence, which is often to say the clash, of expectations between cultures are fully apparent in our hospitals and health science centers. There, the sick and ill fed of alien cultures fetch up soon after their arrival. This is no abstraction. The waves of East Asian citizens who crossed the Pacific after Saigon became Ho Chi Minh City have now reached the staid old cities of the United States' East Coast. There is nothing more readily guaranteed than this unsettled global village to stimulate interest in the background of non-Western medicine.

The immediacy of this problem of medicine and culture brings me to the third approach I mentioned as an expanding one. The borderlands between medical history and a variety of strains of sociology and anthropology seem also due for continued and extended exploration. This is neither a prescription nor a call-to-arms, but simply an observation about a development that is already well under way in what one observer has called the "interpretive turn" in the history of the disciplines.[16] The social scientists are seeing to that. A minority but growing voice among sociologists, in particular, has turned to the historical examination of institutions and systems of health care. Anthropologists evince, on the physical side, a renewed interest in paleopathology, while on the social and cultural front they provide the tools for a more symmetrical approach to understanding therapeutic and hygienic mentalities. Physicians, particularly in the expanding clinical fields devoted to primary care, have begun to learn directly from these new near-neighbors.

So, too, have historians. That this interpretive borderland with the humanistic social sciences should be fertile in the 1980s is suggested by certain of its analytical possibilites and features. For one thing, it becomes possible to talk about innovation, therapeutic or otherwise, without the trappings and celebratory bunting of triumphalist history.[17]

For another, these tools and attitudes allow an interpretive approach that may foster a more fully integrated history of medicine. What would this look like? I take it that such an approach would involve studying the interplay between changing patterns of disease, the medical profession, and theoretical medical science. It would deal with the context of attitudes and structures in which medicine struggles and survives. While it is difficult at this early juncture to exemplify this approach with an entirely satisfactory list of recent work, it seems clear that certain of the efforts of historians like Karl Figlio, Robert Hudson, Guenter Risse, and John Warner on the development of nosology have come encouragingly close.[18]

Such a program would, if successful, avoid the main pitfall that so much of the history of science amd medicine has stumbled into during debates over "internal" versus "external" approaches; namely, that of divorcing context and content. Some medical historians have already begun exploiting its possibilities. If they continue, I think the health science centers will (even more than they already have) sit up and take notice. For it is at this level of integration—with changing patterns of disease, professional interests, and theoretical expertise all laid out complexly in a single tapestry—that the health professions actually *live*. Essentially, then, this interpretive turn in the history of medicine will entail an eclecticism of evidence and explanation that matches the experience of its audience. Increasingly, the medical center audience is becoming precisely the one with the most eclectic and catholic experience.

That audience is also the one that some of us in the history of medicine have begun, ironically, taking for granted. In the past twenty-five years our overall audience has expanded enormously. Some of us, including those of us who began in medicine rather than history, now teach more undergraduate history students than we do medical or paramedical students. Perhaps because the arts curriculum has itself undergone so many changes and adaptations in a quarter century, we have perforce used imagination and experimentation to insure the place of medical history with that other clientele.

By contrast, the medical school curriculum has changed little in seventy-five years. Despite "core" curricula and other "innovations," most changes have been essentially cosmetic, preserving a hierarchy of knowledge that corresponds to now well-entrenched and carefully managed interests. The relationship of the various neighboring disciplines, including medical history, to the overall process has thus become like that of the parts of a foot to an old slipper. (Medical history might be likened to the sixth toe.) Comfort and complacency increase until the whole thing becomes threadbare. Now there are those who are calling for a new shoe, and not primarily because of or for the benefit of a new medical history.[19]

Rather than asking whether the new slipper will fit, I think we as medical historians should be helping to shape the last upon which it will be crafted. It seems a remarkable opportunity. The health professional schools, responding to their own students' concerns, are going to be more and more willing to experiment with "science-plus" curricula. Their students are deeply concerned with the very thing that Jean Starobinski, in his review of Dr. Temkin's *Double Face of Janus,* described as the principal benefit of the history of medicine. "This concern," wrote Starobinski, is not the physician's ideas *per se,* but his *"relationship* with his knowledge," and, one might add, with his clinical behavior and practice.[20] I take it that this is what Howard Mumford Jones meant when he provided his definition of a humane education. "A wise and living scholarship," he said, "is not content with research, it also seeks comprehension, and the freedom to reach comprehension untroubled by the clamors of those who insist that their own view is the only view."[21]

The age-old credo of a liberal education is still serviceable and compelling: an old but still important utility for our discipline. There are new neighbors and new patrons. But one of the oldest patrons—the medical school—may yet again become, in the 1980s, one of the strongest. What remains to be seen is whether we are up to the task.

Notes

1. Thus, research—choice of topic, breadth and depth of penetration, format—is often held unswervingly sacrosanct in the historians' career, while teaching is rather more vulnerable to shifting winds. Hence teaching is more responsive to social and political pressure of a variety of locally and temporally bounded types. Last year the great men and moral uplift; this year ethical perspectives and human values; next year health policy and social engineering.

2. This process has been dubbed "self-exemplification" and discussed by Arnold Thackray and Robert K. Merton, "On discipline-building: the paradoxes of George Sarton," *Isis,* 1972, *63:* 473–95; see also J. R. Cole and Harriet Zuckerman, "The emergence of a scientific specialty: the self-exemplifying case of the sociology of science," in *The Idea of Social Structure: Papers in Honor of Robert K. Merton,* ed. L. A. Coser (New York: Harcourt, Brace, Jovanovich, 1975), pp. 139–74. Also of interest on discipline formation is Charles Rosenberg, "Toward an ecology of knowledge: on discipline, context, and history," in *The Organization of Knowledge in Modern America: 1860–1920,* ed. Alexandra Oleson and John Voss (Baltimore: The Johns Hopkins University Press, 1979), pp. 440–55.

3. The literature on professionalization has become voluminous and will not be summarized here. Four recent monographs that merit attention are: B. J. Bledstein, *The Culture of Professionalism* (New York: W. W. Norton, 1976); Rue Bucher and J. G. Stelling, *Becoming Professional* (Beverly Hills & London: Sage, 1977); Terence Johnson, *Professions and Power* (London: Macmillan, 1972); and M. S. Larson, *The Rise of Professionalism: a Sociological Analysis* (Berkeley: University of California Press, 1977).

4. On the differential uses of the ideal of science in medicine, see R. C. Maulitz, " 'Physician versus bacteriologist': the ideology of science in clinical medicine," in *The Therapeutic Revolution: Essays*

in the Social History of American Medicine, ed. Morris J. Vogel and Charles E. Rosenberg (Philadelphia: University of Pennsylvania Press, 1979), pp. 91–108.

5. George Rosen, "Levels of integration in medical historiography: a review," *J. Hist. Med.,* 1949, *4:* 60–67.

6. Henry Sigerist, "On Hippocrates," in *Henry E. Sigerist on the History of Medicine,* ed. Felix Marti-Ibanez (New York: M.D. Publications, 1960), pp. 97–119.

7. I thank Miss Christine Ruggere, Curator, Historical Collections, College of Physicians of Philadelphia, for useful discussion of this point.

8. After preparation of this chapter I was able to examine the following symposium volume, which is also relevant to the point: J. B. Blake, ed., *Centenary of Index Medicus: 1879–1979* (Washington, D.C.: United States Government Printing Office, 1980); see especially the articles by Charles E. Rosenberg, "Between two worlds: American medicine in 1879," pp. 3–18, and J. B. Blake, "Billings and before: nineteenth century medical bibliography," pp. 31–52.

9. See Maulitz, " 'Physician versus bacteriologist.' "

10. Knud Faber, *Nosography in Modern Internal Medicine* (New York: Hoeber, 1923).

11. Part of this story is available in Arnold Thackray, "The prehistory of an academic discipline: the study of the history of science in the United States, 1891–1941," *Minerva,* 1980, *18:* 448–73.

12. It is not appropriate to attempt here to present a guide to this now voluminous literature as it impinges on medicine and the physician. But see the general observations made by Charles E. Rosenberg in his essay review, "Nature decoded," *Isis,* 1980, *71:* 291–95.

13. John Bostock, *A Sketch of the History of Medicine, from its Origin to the Commencement of the Nineteenth Century* (London: Sherwood, Gilbert, & Piper, 1835), p. 226.

14. Ibid., p. 227.

15. See, for example, Irvine S. L. Loudon and Rosemary Stevens, "Primary care and the hospital," in *Primary Care,* ed. John Fry (London: Heinemann, 1980), pp. 139–75; and W. H. McNeill, *The Human Condition* (Princeton: Princeton University Press, 1980).

16. Clifford Geertz, "Blurred genres," *American Scholar,* spring 1980, pp. 165–79.

17. An example of this approach to the history of therapeutics is Charles E. Rosenberg, "The therapeutic revolution: medicine, meaning, and social change in nineteenth-century America," in Vogel and Rosenberg, *Therapeutic Revolution,* pp. 3–26.

18. Some interesting first approximations of this sort of work are beginning to emerge; see, for example, John Harley Warner, "Therapeutic explanation and the Edinburgh bloodletting controversy: two perspectives on the medical meaning of science in the mid-nineteenth century," *Med. Hist.,* 1980, *24:* 241–58; Guenter B. Risse, "Epidemics and medicine: the influence of disease on medical thought," *Bull. Hist. Med.,* 1979, *53:* 505–19; and two recent articles on chlorosis: Robert Hudson, "The biography of disease: lessons from chlorosis," *Bull. Hist. Med.,* 1977, *51:* 448–63; and Karl Figlio, "Chlorosis and chronic disease in nineteenth-century Britain: the social constitution of somatic illness in a capitalist society," *J. Soc. Hist.,* 1978, *3:* 167–97.

19. Examples of this genre include Carleton B. Chapman, "Should there be a commission on medical education?", *Science,* 1979, *205:* 559–62, and Robert H. Ebert, "Can the education of the physician be made more rational?", *N. Eng. J. Med.,* 1981, *305:* 1343–46.

20. Jean Starobinski's review of Owsei Temkin, *The Double Face of Janus,* in *Bull. Hist. Med.,* 1978, *52:* 281–85; p. 283.

21. Howard Mumford Jones, "The general education stream of the liberal arts," in *What Is a University?* [n.a.] (Cambridge, Mass.: Harvard University Press, 1938?), pp. 32–33.

⍟COMMENTARY

Robert P. Hudson

⍟The principal title of Professor Temkin's immensely useful collected papers, *The Double Face of Janus,* could well have subtitled Dr. Maulitz's present essay.[1] The first section—the backward contemplation—surveys the several fissures, to use the Maulitz metaphor, that developed in the relationship between medical history, medical historians, and medical schools in the nineteenth and first half of the twentieth century. The forward look attempts to identify three major areas in which medical history in the near future will experience different or amplified interactions with what now must be called health professional schools.

Underpinning both the backward and forward observations is the assumption that medical history is unified by an interest in research and teaching, indeed that these two endeavors are inseparable. Since I have argued elsewhere that there is reason to examine the pervasive belief that one cannot be a good teacher without engaging in research, such a definite bonding of these two functions would appear to present an immediate problem for me.[2] Soon after my position on this matter appeared in print, I was approached by Professor Temkin, who began with a gentle questioning as if to be certain he understood my position, but which alerted me, as it probably would have alerted his other students, to the probability that I had suffered some more-or-less monumental lapse of logic. He observed that my position would appear more tenable if I stipulated that the good teacher engages in research as an inescapable part of preparing his instructional presentations, whether he publishes the results or not. I, of course, had neither a way nor desire to debate the now-obvious point, and replied only that I agreed completely and should have said as much in my paper. Dr. Maulitz does not define research, and in any event we are asked only to *assume* with him the identity of research and teaching, so the point need not be belabored further here. His basic aim remains to examine the past, present, and future of medical history, as exemplified by research and teaching, in its relationship to what he terms its patrons and neighbors.

His analysis of the past and present relationships is concise, lucid, and interesting, and I would comment on only one aspect of the story.

The current dialogue, at times heated, concerning what Maulitz calls the "new skepticism" in medical history, I find mostly confusing. And my confusion comes not from his presentation of the schism, but from the very fact and content of the dialogue itself. No one denies that much of the medical history written fifty years ago by practicing physicians was iatrocentric or "internal" as it is called. What is surprising is that these early commentators should be taken to task for their labors at this late date. Their training and outlook dictated such an approach, and it would have been remarkable if they had come at it as social historians or cliometricians. In the same way, I understand those who argue nowadays that the history of medicine can be viewed as a social phenomenon, and that it can illuminate as well as be illuminated by its social context. What I fail to comprehend is why we should pay much attention to the current extremists on this point. I know of no social or nonsocial medical historian who would argue that Pasteur's achievement in discrediting spontaneous generation derived purely from the greatness of the man, and was wholly independent of religious, political, and other social overtones in France at the time. And so I must agree with the recent observation that such attacks simply come a generation too late.[3] In the same vein, I can agree that many social factors influenced the changes of the post-Flexnerian era of American medical education, but I cannot bring myself to bother long with those who, for example, would reduce the importance of Flexner the man to the point of expunging him altogether from the historical record, as was attempted at the last meeting of our association.

It seems unarguable to me that we need to involve all factors: the total constitution of individuals as well as the social forces that aid and restrict human actions. What bothers me is the step that frequently follows, the veiled and not-so-veiled implication that we are somehow derelict because of our particular chosen emphasis. Given the intellectual limitations imposed on most of us, it seems to be inevitable that we would divide the historical labor, with some attacking a given event from its psychological and genetic aspects while others will analyze the political or intellectual or economic forces involved. Only a few, and we will be grateful for them, will rise consistently to the global approach. During the Macy conference on teaching medical history, Genevieve Miller commented candidly on the problem she has in answering medical questions about disease when dealing with a medical audience.[4] I admired her for that admission, and had I been there, I would have confessed my weaknesses in the economic history of the Middle Ages and other deficiencies in social history too abundant to enumerate here.

Maulitz notes, and I believe correctly, that the issue is, in any event, not new in medical history, that we have had our cycles before. We were reminded recently that Shryock's *Development of Modern Medicine* is now more than forty years old.[5] Even the debate is not new. In 1950 Evans-Pritchard was contending that social anthropology was "closer to certain kinds of history than to the natural sciences."[6] In that same year Edwin Boring, the Harvard psychologist, examined the issue in an essay entitled "Great men and scientific progress," in which he concluded that individual human character does count for something in history.[7] Two years before, Aaron Ihde had argued the opposite case in a paper called "The inevitability of scientific discovery."[8]

What is new, and it seems to me, erroneous, is the assumption that either the "external" or "internal" approach to viewing medical history must be wrong. I take it that Maulitz, too, believes there is a place for both, or some amalgam thereof, and that is why he takes heart and predicts that "out of this dialectical process something important survives," and that we will emerge "newly invigorated."

In venturing into the future, Maulitz takes a step historians traditionally have approached with a timidity born of wisdom. He does it, however, largely as a short-range extension of three phenomena he identifies as already operating on the current scene. This is a short step, and one I find justified. In the matter of history and prediction, my position is close to that of Paul Schrecker, who held that even though "the historical disciplines do not pretend to, do not want to, and do not try to predict, they, and they alone, are able to provide the empirical basis for certain sciences of which prediction is expected, namely, certainly all the social sciences, and . . . in some respects also the sciences of nature."[9]

As he surveys the current and future scene, Maulitz identifies three areas in which he sees medical history expanding its efforts in the near future. The first borderland relates to contemporary history. He emphasizes the "tension we feel between the explosiveness and ephemerality of knowledge," and concludes that as these tensions are felt by health professional schools, "it will become a matter of both obligation and equity" for the schools to increase their support of efforts to write contemporary history. Each of us is likely to react to this conclusion in parochial fashion, that is, by testing it against our experience in the one or few schools we know well. As much as I hope Maulitz is correct, when I look at my own institution I come away uncertain at most. The basic scientists and clinicians I know are well aware of, and frequently mention to their students, the fact that knowledge is simultaneously exploding and eroding. They openly paraphrase the nineteenth-century preceptor who told his parting students that he knew that half of what he had taught them was not true, but what disturbed him was that he did not know which half. As nearly as I can detect, my colleagues are scarcely made uncomfortable by this phenomenon, and indeed appear

quite able to ignore it even immediately after calling attention to it. To
this point they have maintained their equanimity by repeatedly sub-
dividing the tree of knowledge to the point that they retain mastery
over an increasingly subspecialized branch—one might even say, twig.
It is possible, and perhaps this is what Maulitz intends, that *outside*
pressures may force them to reexamine their blithe spirits. I have yet to
see much evidence that change will come from their perception of the
matter as a problem demanding examination and action of their own.

The second direction in which Maulitz sees us moving is toward
global history. From a study of the medical history of other cultures he
envisions practical gains for the health schools in dealing with certain of
their own social problems. All would agree, I suppose, that we need to
know more about the medical history of Africa and the East. Further, it
seems highly likely that society generally could benefit from such
endeavors. What the final product would resemble I have trouble visual-
izing. In short, how much would Western medicine change from such
historical assimilation? It would be interesting to know if American
private physicians dealing with individual patients changed their
theories and practices to accommodate the large waves of Oriental and
European immigrants of a century ago. Or did these newcomers, and
the next generation, simply adapt to the existing medical establishment?
Maulitz rightly points out that large numbers of persons are entering our
country at this time, bringing systems of medical belief quite alien to our
own. What I rather imagine is happening, at the moment at least, is that
the West Indian victim of a root, or hex, who presents at a Miami
emergency room, is going home with a prescription for Valium. At the
same time, there is a growing rejection of the human fragmentation that
features current medical education and practice. Whether you spell it
with the *w* or without, the skeletal importance of the wholistic health
movement and the emphasis on family medicine is public disaffection
with the dominant medical system. The extent to which all this will
impinge on academics in ways that will enhance a global view of
medical history can be only a matter of conjecture at this time.

The last category relates to what Maulitz calls "interpretive
history," a term which continues to nag at me a bit in that it has long
been a part of the historian's craft. Insofar as my understanding takes
me, I find myself in nearly complete accord with his thesis. Certainly
there is a large and growing movement now afoot that finds other
disciplines examining the institutions and systems of health care. And
certainly, to the extent that these efforts lead to an increasing tendency
on the part of medical historians to consider context as well as content,
such scrutinies can only be seen as laudable. The degree to which all
this will attract the attention of academic health professionals is, again,
less certain to me. Even though we begin integrating our history in a

fashion that approximates the reality of the health professional's current existence, it does not necessarily follow that they will find us more useful. For this to happen, they will have to be listening to us in the first place—to be at least open to examining the new "interpretive history." In this regard it might be remembered that medicine's altered attitudes toward patient rights, death and dying, and ethical issues in general did not arise from academics *or* private practitioners. The first academic notice of these matters, and the changes that followed, occurred only after a large buildup of public opinion and judicial intervention. Which again is not to say that similar indirect pressures might not produce a greater appreciation by health professionals of the contributions of medical historians and the new interpretive history. In my own institution I see little to suggest any such intramural change within the next decade. But I would benefit greatly from being mistaken on this point, and certainly I would hope with Dr. Maulitz that if it comes, we will be equal to the challenge.

Notes

1. Owsei Temkin, *The Double Face of Janus and Other Essays in the History of Medicine* (Baltimore: Johns Hopkins University Press, 1977).

2. R. P. Hudson, "Goals in the teaching of medical history," *Clio Medica,* 1975, *10:* 156.

3. Lloyd Stevenson, "A second opinion," *Bull. Hist. Med.,* 1980, *54:* 134–40.

4. J. B. Blake, ed., *Education in the History of Medicine* (New York: Hafner Publishing, 1968), p. 71.

5. Stevenson, "Second opinion," p. 138.

6. E. E. Evans-Pritchard, *Anthropology and History* (Manchester: The University Press, 1961), p. 1.

7. E. G. Boring, "Great men and scientific progress," *Proc. Am. Phil. Soc.,* 1950, *94:* 339–51.

8. A. J. Ihde, "The inevitability of scientific discovery," *Sci. Monthly,* 1948, *67:* 427–29.

9. P. Schrecker, "Historians, empiricists, and prophets," in *On the Utility of Medical History,* ed. I. Galdston (New York: International Universities Press, 1957), pp. 72–73.

ANTECEDENTS TO CONTEMPORARY HEALTH ISSUES: HISTORY, POLITICS, AND THE POLICY OF HEALTH

Arthur J. Viseltear

The presentations we hear today are personal histories. Each discussed is a glimpse of one's career which, as with life itself, is often dependent upon a confluence of educational experiences, academic exigencies, historical accident, and personal choice. The course I tell you about today, then, is as much about me as it is about the nature of the Yale curriculum in which it is placed.

I. In a more tumultuous time in American history, Henry E. Sigerist addressed the Third Eastern Medical Students Conference. Some three hundred medical students and faculty members from fifteen different medical schools assembled in New Haven in 1936 to discuss the rapid changes then occurring in society and medical practice. "Time marches on inexorably," he said. "There is no way back. There is but one way for us to go, the way that leads into the future." [1] Sigerist cited contemporary problems, including war, hunger, disease, and the high cost of medical care. He discussed comparative national systems of medical care and lamented the fact that many in our country did not receive adequate health care and that many died prematurely. If the medical conditions were not satisfactory they should be changed, he said. And how should the "young generation" go about resolving these social and medical problems? By the study of history, political economy, and sociology. History "teaches us where we stand today and what tasks have been assigned to us." It also makes "unconscious trends conscious so that we can face and discuss them openly." [2]

Sigerist told the students that he was addressing these issues in a "sociological course" in which he traced the development and interrelationships of society and the medical profession. In this course, he considered the changing nature of medical practice over time, medical services in ancient societies, medical organizations in feudal societies, the rise of capitalism, the industrial revolution and its consequences for the health of the populace, socialized medicine in Germany, the political philosophies of liberalism, fascism, and socialism, and the American situation, including medical economic surveys and contemporary experiments in the organization, delivery, and financing of health services.[3] He said most schools were beginning to recognize that students should have some instruction in this area but that most did it in a haphazard way. Little emphasis was given to health services research, medical sociology, or medical economics. Perhaps the social and economic implications of medicine could be examined in a separate department of the medical school, but, in the interim, his immediate message was to read (newspapers, journals of opinion, novels, and the classics), to discuss (topics of contemporary importance, such as housing, preventive medicine, the social aspects of communicable diseases, municipal public health problems, and even the recent neutrality legislation), and to speak out.[4] "Remember," he said in his conclusion, "you cannot afford to stand aside. . . . [you must] make an effort to understand the foundation of our society, to analyze the tendencies and trends."[5]

Professor Sigerist's exhortation was heeded by many in the late 1930s and 1940s. Medical students and medical school graduates, in various publications and before various audiences, considered a host of social issues, including the need for federal social insurance programs. Many dedicated, energetic, and socially motivated physicians gravitated to Washington during the war years, seeking careers in public service and involvement in federal programs concerned with rural and migrant health, communicable disease control, medical care, and state health services. Many prepared memoranda, wrote speeches, engaged in health services research, prepared medical economic health surveys, or collected and collated health statistics and epidemiologic data. Some became members of the American Public Health Association, joining the Health Administration or Epidemiology Sections and then coming together in common purpose to establish a new Section on Medical Care.[6] Others involved themselves in the Physician's Forum or the Association of Interns and Medical Students.[7]

The common bond uniting these young crusaders was Sigerist. Some were captivated by his scholarship, charm, and urbanity, but mostly all, having lived through the Depression and seeing for themselves conditions existing in rural America, the inner city, and in county or municipal hospitals, recognized at once the clarity and purpose of Sigerist's message. These were no mindless automatons listening to a siren song; rather they were critical young men and women already imbued with a purpose, in Sigerist's words, "to accelerate . . . developments [that would] make this world a better world."[8]

One of Sigerist's students was Milton Roemer, who, after work with Joseph Mountin in the Federal Security Agency, public health work in Morgantown, West Virginia, consultantships in the World Health

Organization and the Saskatchewan Provincial Government, came to UCLA as professor of medical care organization.

Concurrent to my work leading to the doctorate in history at UCLA, I was able to enroll in a number of Dr. Roemer's seminars and eventually to see that my own career lay not in studies of eighteenth-century medicine and therapeutics but in contemporary history.[9] This was a troubling decision because the recent past was often dismissed with the disparaging comment that it was not really history but "journalism." Professor Roemer, reliving his own experiences with Sigerist, however, believed just the opposite. Contemporary history was a necessity because the present and future could only be understood by studying the past.[10] Study the past, he said, not only for its own sake but for how it bears on contemporary problems and dilemmas. If you have a choice, he seemed to be saying, become "present minded" and not "history minded."[11]

Despite this suggestion, I found myself interested not so much in the present as in the past. Placing oneself too near an issue of burning contemporary importance did not lead to dispassionate analysis, I felt, and so, when hired by the School of Public Health to prepare case studies of contemporary medical care topics, I avoided the present as best I could and instead concerned myself, as would any journeyman historian, with the memos, transcripts, minutes, letters, and diaries found in various archival depositories. The case studies I prepared would be methodologically sound and historically impeccable. My narratives would not be polemics, but rigorous analyses based on fact.

The case studies we prepared at UCLA (analyzing, for example, the decision to build a hospital in Watts, the dissolution of the osteopathic profession in California, and the early years of the Ross-Loos Medical Clinic) proved to be valuable teaching aids. In preparing them I had gone back in time; in class, however, the instructor went forward. The operative questions were: "What can we learn from this case? How can we use the information provided to help us with our present-day concerns?" And the students oddly never seemed to lack answers.

II. Arriving at Yale in 1969, I was soon caught up with a need to be contemporary. Here I was collegially associated with George Rosen, George Silver, E. Richard Weinerman, and Isidore Falk, each a student or associate of Sigerist's. Here, too, was Rosemary Stevens, then completing her manuscript of *American Medicine and the Public Interest.* I was hired to teach a section of the introductory medical care course and to offer a seminar on the History of Social Insurance, but I sought also to bring historical method to bear, as Rosemary Stevens was doing, to contemporary health care issues. Together with George Rosen and another Yale colleague, Dr. Stevens and I developed a proposal for a History and

Health Policy Research Unit in the medical school. Using the combined methodologies and skills of historians and policy analysts, went our argument, would permit present-day analysts to advance more efficiently and accurately health policy determination, formulation, and innovation. We were to be especially concerned with how and why, and with what implications, health policies, programs, and legislation had been designed and translated into action. Unhappily, the proposal never emerged from the draft memorandum stage, but it did help to advance the idea within my parent Department of Epidemiology and Public Health that the subject matter was worthy of continued consideration.

In 1974, I was awarded a Robert Wood Johnson Health Policy Fellowship which brought me to Washington, D.C., for a year of seminar and congressional assignment. Here I found that I was in the center of an odd universe, learning to understand and mistrust power, examining others' and my own ambitions and motives, and learning also to appreciate the anguish and ambiguity of compromise. This was a heady and intoxicating experience but, as the year progressed, I found myself reacting to the players and the process as had Doris Kearns, "with alternating awe, admiration, fascination, fear, and disdain." [12] So, after formulating policy, playing with budgets in the megamillions, writing speeches, orchestrating hearings—in short, after finding myself in an arena in which I myself had become a player in history—I returned to the university to resume my research and teaching.

I found that I was much in demand to share my observations and experiences with my colleagues and students. I was placed on the medical-school Planning and Priorities Committee, elected to the medical school council, and invited to speak at colloquia and classes in my parent and other departments and at the Institution for Social and Policy Studies (ISPS). Before the council, I discussed the manpower legislation, which in 1976 had become for many university presidents, including Yale's Kingman Brewster and Johns Hopkins's Stephen Muller, "that wretched business." I considered the current drug reform bill at a colloquium sponsored by the Department of Pharmacology, discussed the new health promotion and preventive medicine legislation from inception to enactment at ISPS, and attempted to define, before a session of the Planning and Priorities Committee, Congress's professed role as "steward of the American people," a role increasingly in conflict with special-interest groups, including the academic medical center. [13] I revised the seminar courses I offered in my parent department and developed a "History and Health Policy" elective that I hoped to offer to medical students. In short, as a result of these activities, I found myself increasingly being pushed not into contemporary history, but into contemporary politics. And I did not resist. Why? Because (in 1975 when I returned) there was a need for someone in the medical school to consider this subject area and because Yale was beginning to recognize at last that it no longer had the luxury of remaining hidden in its ivy fortress, eschewing both politics and reality. As Robert Petersdorf has recently written, "The days of splendid isolation from the world are gone forever. Academic medicine is very much in the public sector, and it demands a new and additional role of all within it—that of the informed, thoughtful academic citizen." [14] And this became my role at Yale.

I had taught medical students before, but despite the fact that my parent department was both a school of public health as well as a department of the medical school, I had not ventured into the medical school (except for the brief experience of teaching George Rosen's course in the history of medicine when he was on sabbatical leave in 1972). In 1975, I wanted very much to offer medical students a seminar course in health policy and petitioned the medical school curriculum committee for time to do so. The committee, which resembles in both demeanor and style a latter-day Grendel, declared that the topic was of insufficient moment to add to Yale's already plethoric curriculum. I asked if I could offer the course on an ad hoc basis, perhaps in the evening, to anyone who showed up and, after some bickering (not about the syllabus but about security for female students attending a course which met in the evening) I was permitted to proceed.

Fifteen medical students and three Robert Wood Johnson Clinical Scholars responded to my memorandum inviting students to join a seminar in which I would discuss the health establishment, medical manpower, preventive medicine, the 1971 National Cancer Act, alternative health care systems, reform of the Food and Drug Administration, clinical laboratories, and national health insurance. The objective was to examine both the history of the policy, program, or legislative initiative and its politics.

Despite its anomalous origins, the course, which was presented under the title, "History, Politics, and the Policy of Health," eventually became part of the formal medical school curriculum in 1978, as an eight-week module of the core course offered to second year students in the medical school by the Department of Epidemiology and Public Health. Under this sponsorship, thirty students asked to participate in the policy module, but only fifteen were admitted in order to distribute students evenly among the other modules.

Concurrent to these activities, following George Rosen's death in 1977, the courses in medical history which he offered in Yale College and the medical school became my responsibility.[15] Professor Rosen was a dedicated and enthusiastic teacher and distinguished scholar who had great success with the course he offered in Yale College. Building upon the popularity of the subject area established by Lloyd Stevenson and Peter Niebyl, Professor Rosen filled his lecture hall with over 100 students in each semester in which the course was offered. The medical school course, however, was less popular with the medical students, for whom all courses are electives and treated as such. Yale began to tinker with its curriculum in the 1960s. The result was to expand the number of hours for such subjects as cell biology, molecular biophysics and biochemistry, and physiology at the expense of gross anatomy, pathology, and the history of medicine. What in the 1950s and 1960s at Yale was a leisurely, eighteen-hour trot through history from antiquity to the present became a 100-meter dash as the course was reduced to eight, one-hour sessions in the 1970s.

Modifying Dr. Rosen's eight-hour course slightly, I included in 1978 the following lecture topics: an introduction and overview of the practice of medicine, archaic medicine, medieval medicine; William Harvey; changing theories of the etiology, prevention, and cure of diseases; medicine in America; a review of health legislation affecting medical practice over the last 100 years; and the rise of modern medicine. A year later, I modified the course to include topics on the scientific revival, the scientific foundation of medicine, and antecedents to contemporary health issues.

The course description for both years described its focus as "A history of the ideas, attitudes, and institutions of medicine from antiquity to modern times, with especial consideration of changing social, economic, and cultural relationships, and of principal players." Listed under various topic headings, students found the following phrases: "The physician in modern society," "Current issues and problems," and "Trends in medical practice." The final, summary lecture in the 1979 course appeared under the title, "History, Politics, and the Policy of Health," as follows:

> Antecedents to contemporary problems. Medical practice. Hospitals and the academic medical center. Changing patterns in the organization, delivery, and financing of health care. The federal government and medicine: a century of concern and tension. Legacies, players and issues revisited.

The course was surprisingly well attended and favorably reviewed by the students. Encouraged by the reception, I requested that the curriculum committee consider expanding the course by a half-semester, thereby restoring the course to its original eighteen hours. I argued that the Yale Corporation had just established a Section of the History of Medicine, that lectures could be added on topics for which there was no opportunity to discuss or only to gloss over, that there was an interest attested to by increased enrollment, and that with the added half-semester the section (Professor F. L. Holmes and myself) could more leisurely and comprehensively peruse our subject rather than have to discuss, for example, Hippocrates and Galen in a single hour.[16]

The request was denied. Having to establish priorities among many competing basic-science interests, they told me, and bound to the principle of reserving unscheduled free time, they could not in good faith expand the history of medicine to a half-semester. The question then asked regarded the module I was then offering in the public health course. Why not extract this module, which they said was "necessary" for all medical students, and offer it as an elective to follow the history of medicine lectures? Despite my protest that the eighteen-hour course envisioned was designed to make room for additional lectures in ancient, Renaissance, seventeenth-, eighteenth-, and early twentieth-century medicine, they merely repeated the question, agreed among themselves that the idea was brilliant, and ultimately approved their own suggestion. (It is just such exquisite nonsense which makes legends of curriculum committees!)

III. This hybrid course, offered for the first time in January 1980, has two discrete but interrelated parts. Part 1 is an "Introduction to Medical History" and begins in antiquity and ends with the Flexner Report in 1910. Part 2, "History, Politics, and the Policy of Health," includes these subject headings: the health establishment, medical manpower, the pharmaceutical industry, biomedical research, medical technology, swine influenza, prevention, national health insurance, and medicine in the 1980s.

The description for the first eight lectures of part 1 remained the same:

A history of the ideas, attitudes, and institutions of medicine from antiquity to the present with especial consideration of changing social, economic, and political factors, and of principal players.

And, the description for the second nine hours reads:

A review of the legislative and executive branches of government and their involvement in the design and implementation of health policy. Specifically, a consideration of antecedents to contemporary health issues, executive and congressional branch policies and tensions and selected congressional legislative initiatives.

Part 2, then, considers American health policy in the present century. I present a number of selected issues of contemporary interest within a framework that is both historical and political, considering origins (or policy genesis), principal and secondary players involved, the culture and unique personality of the federal bureaucracy, the strategies and ploys associated with the development and enactment of the program, the roles of congressional staff, academic consultants, science advisers, the media and lobbyists, and the interlocking complexities of political reality.[17]

The approach is similar for each case presented. In considering medical manpower, for example, I begin with a review of eighteenth- and nineteenth-century medical practice, irregular medicine, the emergence of the "new science," the rise of specialism, indications of manpower shortages as reported in various foundation or federal health surveys, and federal legislative initiatives from the 1960s to the present. I address specialty and geographic maldistribution, dependence on foreign medical graduates, and selected congressional concerns regarding primary care, curriculum innovation, and scholarships and loan support. And in an epilogue to the 1980 lecture, I considered the growing evidence and implications of a doctor surplus, recently set forth by the Graduate Medical Education National Advisory Committee.

A review of the pharmaceutical industry begins with the climate of opinion, state of therapeutic and medical knowledge, legislative responses, and impact of selected legislative proposals dating from 1906. From congressional hearings and reports, transcripts of debates appearing in the *Congressional Record,* and selected secondary source readings, the topics I consider include drug efficacy, economics, the role of detail-men, advertising, generic versus trade names, the role of the Pharmaceutical Manufacturers Association and other interest groups, the testimony of witnesses, the questions asked by Congressional Committee members, the apologias of agency chiefs, a statement about present and future prospects, and an institutional profile of the Food and Drug Administration.[18]

Another case is national health insurance, the origins of which I trace to the Marine Hospital Service, social insurance in Germany and Great Britain, workmen's compensation, the American Association for Labor Legislation, state medicine in Russia, the early, abortive legislative attempts of the "almost persuaded generation," the genesis, activities, and impact of the Committee on the Costs of Medical Care, Edgar Sydenstricker, John A. Kingsbury, C.-E. A. Winslow, the "lost reform" of 1935, the role of the American Medical Association, the activities of the Technical Committee, the National Health Conference, and the insurgent Committee of Physicians for the Improvement of Medical Care, John P. Peters, Alan Butler, Channing Frothingham, the social insurance programs proposed in the 1930s and 1940s, Michael M. Davis, Josephine Roche, Martha Eliot, Henry Sigerist, I. S. Falk, Joseph Mountin, the "100 Percenters," Kerr-Mills, King-Anderson, Medicaid, HMOs, and Kennedy-Griffiths and Kennedy-Mills to today's catastrophic and consumer choice alternatives.[19]

Topics considered in the first eight hours of the course referred to in this lecture include state health services in Greece, municipal physicians in Rome, physician reimbursement in various time periods, John Bellars, friendly societies, Lord Dawson of Penn, regionalization, and charity, dispensary, and hospital care at the turn of the century.[20]

Similar historical linkages and associations are made in other lectures as well. Biomedical research, for example, considers the emergence in America of a scientific establishment, the research environment necessary for science to thrive, and the present controversies over budgets, priorities, consumer concerns, and congressional oversight.[21] Prevention considers how the spore of prevention, after a prolonged absence, has recently reestablished itself in fertile soil.[22] Is prevention a litany of the obvious, the new magic, an answer to our present health care dilemmas?[23] Is it cost effective?[24] Does it work? Is the surgeon-general's report conclusive?[25] And what about swine influenza? Is this case representative of scientific decisionmaking? Is the lesson to be learned that too much rather than too little attention was paid to history? Could anything have been learned from a review of other mass immunization programs, such as polio or measles? Are elements of confusion, stupidity, and cognitive dissonance a norm or unique to this case?[26]

In the concluding lecture I consider the present state of medicine. Flexner is revisited, the trilateral relationship of government, the academic medical center, and the consumer is discussed as is the federal budget.[27] I review the life and times of two quasi-fictitious practitioners who graduated medical school in 1932 and 1944, and consider increasing consumer demands and sophistication and regulatory politics and economics.[28] There is also an epilogue in which I present certain personal observations selected from the historical medical literature revealing that physicians marry, have children, and occasionally divorce, are not without a sense of humor, write novels, essays, and poetry, lead rich or humdrum lives, are often politically astute and active, and eventually grow old, get sick, and die.[29]

IV. The entire course of seventeen hours considers medicine, society, and politics. It is markedly different from other courses in the history of medicine. At the same time it is also derivative as it is based upon courses that have considered the physician in society, a subject that came to be called "medical care" and that, outside of Johns Hopkins in the 1930s and early 1940s, was found primarily in schools of public health offered by instructors who well understood the organizational and financial issues attendant to medical care and appreciated the value of considering present problems by examining the historical record of past achievements and failures.[30] Many of these instructors, after all, had been associated with the Committee on the Costs of Medical Care, and others had been students of Henry Sigerist.[31]

As with all electives, the future of these two half-semester courses is dependent upon a host of factors, not the least of which happens to be student and faculty interest, which is often fickle, short lived, and difficult to fathom.[32] I expect the syllabus of this nascent course to change, perhaps to become the consolidated "History of Medicine" course as originally planned, or to go off in another, related direction, as a "History of Medical Care." Its dual focus on the past and present, and how the past influences the present, however, will remain the same. By choice and character, perhaps also by accident, this is the course that I have come to offer at Yale.

Notes

1. H. E. Sigerist, "The medical student and the social problems confronting medicine today," *Bull. Hist. Med.*, 1936, *4:* 411.

2. Ibid., pp. 415–16.

3. Ibid., pp. 418–19.

4. Ibid., p. 420.

5. Ibid., p. 422.

6. See A. J. Viseltear, *Emergence of the Medical Care Section of the American Public Health Association, 1926–1948: A Chapter in the History of Medical Care* (Washington, D.C.: American Public Health Association, 1972); see also M. I. Roemer, "The American Public Health Association as a force for change in medical care," *Medical Care*, 1973, *11:* 338–51.

7. See, for example, *Report of the Conference on the Problems of Medical Care, Washington, D.C., December 8–9, 1944* (New York: Physician's Forum, 1944); for information about AIMS, see issues of *The Intern*, their official organ.

8. Sigerist, "Medical student," p. 422.

9. A. J. Viseltear, "The lithontriptic medicines of the eighteenth century" (Ph.D. diss.: UCLA, 1965). In 1960, I enrolled in a newly established doctoral program in history. Established by C. D. O'Malley and A. Rupert Hall at UCLA, the program called for fields in the history of medicine, the history of science, history, and an allied science. Concurrent with my studies for the Ph.D. (awarded in 1965), I was able to obtain an M.P.H. degree (in 1963) as I pursued course work in public health, the subject area of my fifth field, the allied science.

10. M. I. Roemer, ed., *Henry E. Sigerist on the Sociology of Medicine* (New York: MD Publications, 1960), pp. xi–xiii.

11. J. H. Hexter, "The historian and his day," in his *Reappraisals in History: New Views on History and Society in Early Modern Europe* (New York: Harper Torchbooks, 1963), pp. 1–4.

12. Doris Kearns, "Angles of vision," in *Telling Lives: The Biographer's Art*, ed. Marc Pachter (Washington, D.C.: New Republic Books, 1979), p. 95.

13. U.S., Congress, Senate, *Health Professions Educational Assistance Act of 1974*, Report No. 93–1133, 3 September 1974 (Washington, D.C.: U.S. Government Printing Office, 1974), p. 212.

14. R. G. Petersdorf, "The academic in Washington—worthwhile effort or waste of time?," *Pharos*, summer 1979, p. 8. For similar views, see P. E. Dans, "Physicians and health policy," *J.A.M.A.*, 1980, *243:* 1451–53, and Rashi Fein, "Medicine and government," *New Eng. J. Med.*, 1980, *303:* 219–21.

15. See A. J. Viseltear, "George Rosen (June 23, 1910–July 27, 1977)," *Yale. J. Biol. Med.*, 1977, *50:* 537–42.

16. See "Appointments in the history of medicine: Yale University," *Bull. Hist. Med.*, 1979, *53:* 300–302.

17. Harold Seidman, *Politics, Position, and Power: The Dynamics of Federal Organization* (New York: Oxford University Press, 1970), p. viii; A. P. Sindler, ed., *American Political Institutions and Public Policy: Five Contemporary Studies* (Boston: Little, Brown, 1969), p. v.

18. R. K. Huitt, "The congressional committee: a case study" in *Congress: Two Decades of Analysis*, ed. R. K. Huitt and R. L. Peabody (New York: Harper & Row, 1969), pp. 77–112.

19. See R. L. Numbers, *Almost Persuaded: American Physicians and Compulsory Health Insurance, 1912–1920* (Baltimore: The Johns Hopkins University Press, 1978); D. S. Hirshfield, *The Lost Reform: The Campaign for Compulsory Health Insurance in the United States from 1932 to 1943* (Cambridge: Harvard University Press, 1970); and see the two-part article by A. C. Enthoven, "Consumer-choice health plan," *New Eng. J. Med.*, 1978, *298*: 650–58, 709–20.

20. A. G. Woodhead, "The state health service in Ancient Greece," *Cambridge Historical J.*, 1952, *10*: 235–53; M. M. Davis, *Clinics, Hospitals and Health Centers* (New York: Harper & Brothers, 1927).

21. See, for example, Marjorie Sun, "Scientists and Congress battle over NIH," *Science*, 1980, *209*: 1497–98; J. R. Krevans, "NIH: handle with care," *New Eng. J. Med.*, 1980, *303*: 45–47; D. S. Greenberg, "NIH: with friends like that . . . ," ibid., 1980, *302*: 1490–92; D. S. Fredrickson, "Health and the search for new knowledge," *Daedalus*, 1977, *106*: 159–70; and Lewis Thomas, *Aspects of Biomedical Science Policy: An Occasional Paper*, Institute of Medicine, National Academy of Sciences (Washington, D.C.: National Academy of Sciences, 1972).

22. George Rosen, *Preventive Medicine in the United States, 1900–1975: Trends and Interpretations* (New York: Science History Publications, 1975); A. J. Viseltear, "Health education and public policy: a short history of P.L. 94–317," in *Preventive Medicine U.S.A.: Task Force Reports Sponsored by the John E. Fogarty International Center for Advanced Study in the Health Sciences, National Institutes of Health, and The American College of Preventive Medicine* (New York: Prodist, 1976), pp. 825–37.

23. Lewis Thomas, "On magic in medicine," *New Eng. J. Med.*, 1978, *299*: 461–63.

24. See J. R. Lave et al., "Economic impact of preventive medicine," in *Preventive Medicine U.S.A.*, pp. 675–714, and R. M. Scheffler and Lynn Paringer, "A review of the economic evidence on prevention," *Medical Care*, 1980, *18*: 473–84.

25. U.S., Department of Health, Education, and Welfare, *Healthy People: The Surgeon General's Report on Health Promotion and Disease Prevention, 1979* (Washington, D.C.: U.S. Government Printing Office, 1979); see also Marc Lalonde, *A New Perspective on the Health of Canadians: A Working Document* (Ottawa: Information Canada, 1975).

26. R. E. Neustadt and H. V. Fineberg, *The Swine Flu Affair: Decision-Making on a Slippery Disease* (Washington, D.C.: U.S. Government Printing Office, 1978); A. J. Viseltear, "Immunization and public policy: a short political history of the 1976 swine influenza legislation," in *Influenza in America, 1918–1976*, ed. June Osborn (New York: Prodist, 1977), pp. 29–58.

27. D. E. Rogers, *American Medicine: Challenge for the 1980s* (Cambridge, Mass.: Ballinger Publishing, 1978).

28. Anne Somers, "Dr. Smith and Dr. Jones: two portraits," in *Health and Health Care: Policies in Perspective*, ed. A. R. Somers and H. M. Somers (Germantown, Md.: Aspen Systems Corporation, 1977), pp. 21–26; Arthur Levin, ed., *Regulating Health Care: The Struggle for Control* (New York: Academy of Political Science, 1980).

29. Many of the excerpts are selected from George Rosen and Beate Caspari-Rosen, *Four Hundred Years of a Doctor's Life* (New York: Henry Schuman, 1947).

30. C.-E. A. Winslow offered one such course as early as 1932 at Yale. See Winslow MSS in Yale's "Contemporary Medical Care and Health Policy Collection."

31. See "A farewell dinner for Dr. and Mrs. Henry E. Sigerist," *Bull. Hist. Med.*, 1948, *22*: 5–46, and Susan Reverby and Davis Rosner, *Health Care in America: Essays in Social History* (Philadelphia: Temple University Press, 1979), p. 9.

32. The Section of the History of Medicine offers other medical school electives and, as well, courses in Yale College and the Graduate School. In the medical school, Professor Holmes and I offer a readings and discussion course on historical medical classics. Other electives include a History of Biochemistry, a History of Anatomy (offered by Professor Thomas Forbes), and a History of Public Health. Section faculty offer in Yale College courses on "The Scientific Foundations of Medicine" and an "Introduction to the History of Medicine." In the Graduate School are offered seminars on "The History of Biology" and "The History of American Medicine and Public Health."

COMMENTARY

Barbara Gutmann Rosenkrantz

Arthur Viseltear enriched his paper with autobiography and it seems reasonable to view his concerns as exemplary. No wonder his ambivalence since the historian's effort to create a single course or a more ambitious curriculum for students in the health professions is often foiled by Grendel, followed closely by the Mad Hatter and the Red Queen. Lucky the "medical teaching center" where this produces a suppressed giggle exploding into a lively course rather than resentment!

There are many reasons why the historian is not given high priority in educating physicians and health scientists and surely it is prudent to look beyond the obvious limitations set by crowded academic schedules. If forced feeding is not recommended, no matter how wholesome the fare, alternatives may be identified. Let us acknowledge the obstacles implicated by Viseltear before proposing new directions: first, the hazards to education (as distinct from training) endemic to professional schools; and second, the treacherous nature of contemporary history. Viseltear's adventures indicate that it would be wise not to underestimate the dangers faced by academic historians in the culture of the medical center. Historians are predictably uneasy with the prospect of "adaptation" or even "cooptation" in professional schools, especially where the liberal arts curriculum has not promoted much innovation. The historian with degree in hand is, understandably, responsive to the traditional academic hierarchy in which the liberal arts reign. Although adversary relationships of graduate and professional school can be exaggerated, the cultural differences are substantial and not resolved by repeating our commitment to the standards of excellence held by disciplinary peers, however praiseworthy this sentiment. Moreover, there are no obvious criteria for evaluating the "middle range" history course designed to meet the intellectual needs of advanced students in the health professions. In this situation "service" courses multiply to fit schedules rather than students. Historians are well aware that the preeminent task of instruction in medical history since the turn of the century has been "socialization" or negotiation between cultures, most often on the sturdy wheels of the survey course.

The alternative offering is contemporary history often based on establishing the linkages of medicine and its allies. But most historians approach the recent past apologetically as though it were not quite clean and certainly not respectable. When the survey course emphasizes connections between the past and present it, too, faces the danger of being "ahistorical," and Viseltear sees the tenderfoot making a forced choice between the present minded and the history minded. These dilemmas have a common ground in insecurity; for most historians, to be scorned as present minded is to forfeit credibility if not credentials at the next professional gathering.

Over the past half-century, historians have been curiously eager to renounce the crime of passion identified by Herbert Butterfield as "Whig history," exemplified by "the tendency . . . to praise revolutions provided they have been successful, to emphasize certain principles of progress in the past and to produce a story which is the ratification if not the glorification of the present."[1] Historians of science and medicine may feel particularly vulnerable to this charge, but it is most certain that the dangers of losing historical perspective cannot be avoided by simply concentrating on the remote rather than the more accessible past.[2] And yet, contemporary history involves most difficult problems. Judicious choice of subject, selection of evidence that living witnesses can appear to contradict, arguments that are simultaneously blessed by scholarly dispassion and appropriate compassion for the conflicts faced by one's students. Absent the capacity of Sigerist, teaching contemporary history requires a rigorous structure in which there is a conscious interchange of expert status between the instructor and the class. Contemporary history purveyed through lecture inevitably solicits a parade of visiting firemen; the seminar requires the discipline and time few students can command. Rarely does the historian feel competent guiding such a seminar since most of us are not particularly familiar with the social sciences that traditionally analyze and interpret recent history.

Nor have historians teaching in schools of medicine and public health found the subject matter or methods of economic and social-science history particularly congenial. Sometimes a colleague health economist or medical sociologist has "covered" the relevant courses and questions, and at other times the historian has eased out of trouble by describing the general economic, political, or social context in which the event of particular concern took shape. A wide variety of absolutely first rate courses have thus well served several generations of students. It is as important to recognize this as it is to be forthright about the frustrations. The perplexities of curriculum committees are not usually generated by instruction in history. Versatile accommodations to reality reflect, moreover, changes in teaching the clinical and science-based curriculum as much as the development of historical research. The intellectual objectives of current trends in the social and biological sciences are also important to historians of medicine, as was the emphasis on the laboratory to reorienting history of medicine at the turn of the century.

I will conclude with brief comments on three issues: the audience we as historians of medicine address, the subject matter of our courses, and the object of teaching the history of medicine to students in the health professions. Because we are not teaching future historians we frequently conclude that our courses should be angled in some unusual way that needs defense or appeal. In part this is a reaction to the uneasy position of history in the curriculum: a course that is open to all comers and designed to awaken interest as much as to satisfy it. Although compulsory enrollment is rare, the course is ordinarily and deliberately accessible to every student qualified to enter medical school; I doubt there is a prerequisite for any course in history. But I would argue that there are students in schools of public health for whom history is essential, and this may well be equally true for some medical students. For instance, the methods and research findings of historical demography are significant to epidemiologists who evaluate the health status of developing nations where the impact of the demographic transition on the incidence of contagious disease can be compared with the history of patterns in highly industrialized nations. Sound historical knowledge as well as sophisticated quantitative analysis is necessary for this research to be appropriately incorporated to the education of health professionals; interpretation of "results" demands judgment based on historical documentation.[3] And "electing" this course in history has quite different implications from choosing the usual elective survey course. If this area of historical studies is included in the curriculum, it may well lead to a new claim on historians that would complement the focus on medical concepts, institutions, and policies.

This approach leads to a selection of students with preparation and interests in the population sciences and epidemiology, but there is no necessary limit based on addressing these substantive questions. The subject matter for historians of medicine includes all aspects of human experience associated with the relationship of health and disease, and the intent of my suggestion is to shift some weight from extensive to intensive coverage. I would take advantage of the difference between history *of* medicine and history *in* medicine.[4] The subject matter for history in medicine is similar to the subject of medical inquiry, based on assumptions similar to those of nineteenth-century historians who announced that medicine was of necessity a social science.[5] One might say that this study is directed to understanding the historical conditions that created symptoms rather than diagnoses. One could select the same event to study from several different viewpoints in order to emphasize these differences between history *of* and history *in* medicine. On the one hand, the case of Typhoid Mary could be investigated through George Soper's accounts and analyses of the scientific, economic, and political variables that created medical and social crises. Alternatively, a model for differential risk from typhoid and diphtheria carriers could be constructed, analyzed, and used in comparing the influences of "biological" and "social" factors in responses of the New York City population to quarantine regulations. Both of these are approaches to understanding a critical event with implications for health professionals, but each method and interpretation has distinct objectives. Both courses, in part because they concentrate on extracting a series of questions from the circumstances of a single event, require that the student be more engaged with history than many health professionals are willing or able to be. In practice this history succeeds best when the student has a foundation of knowledge in the biomedical and social sciences, and by that criterion alone infers a professional objective.

Viseltear's chapter and my comments both take for granted that the merit of historical study is judged by its value to the student. The response to Sigerist in the 1930s reflected a meeting of talent and circumstance in what Viseltear calls "a tumultuous time" when students felt compelled to examine the past as a guide to the future. Identification of crises is an occupational hazard for historians, but it is my sense that each generation finds its own sense of destiny, and that students preparing for the health professions today are also very much preoccupied with their social role. One traditional function of historical studies is to "provide perspective," and this seems to be equally true for students in professional schools. The perspective here is necessarily at odds with that of the introductory college course, since professional students have already made commitments that place them as specialists in relation to their own past status as undergraduate generalists. The value of history for them may be to place this commitment in a larger context and to provide experience with the tools historians take for granted. In addition to the survey course, a literature review on a specific topic would serve them well, as would the opportunity to use historical resources and methods rather than being limited to secondary materials.

What is my own measure of success as a teacher? The altered expectation that is evident when I no longer hear the question most frequently asked at the beginning of the course: what is the right answer? Instead I hope to transmit a conviction that what you ask of the past, and how you ask, determines what you will study and understand. Obviously Viseltear and I follow different strategies toward a common goal. In his writing, as in his teaching, he uses wry humor to close the gap between the historian and the health professional. I have learned from Viseltear as well. Since my foremost objective in teaching is to provoke critical and informed response to conventional wisdom, my purposes might best be served if I simply stood beside an artifact from contemporary history—the handsome poster of the 1960s in which a silent Buddha presides over the caption, "Don't just go out and do something—sit there."

Notes

1. *The Whig Interpretation of History* (London: M. Bell, 1931), p. v.

2. David L. Hull, "In defense of presentism," *History and Theory*, 1979, *18:* 1–15.

3. The potential for "a new antiquarianism" based on numerical data is, of course, no less than the potential for the more familiar antiquarianism that historians of medicine have always resisted.

4. For an interesting discussion of the background to this distinction in sociology, see Linda H. Aiken and Howard E. Freeman, "Medical sociology and science and technology in medicine," in *A Guide to the Culture of Science, Technology, and Medicine,* ed. Paul T. Durbin (New York: Free Press, 1980), p. 531.

5. George Rosen, "What is social medicine? a genetic analysis of the concept," *Bull. Hist. Med.,* 1947, *21:* 674–733, especially sections I–III.

PHARMACEUTICAL HISTORY FOR THE PHARMACY STUDENT

John Parascandola

Although the main purpose of this paper is to discuss the teaching of the history of pharmacy at the University of Wisconsin, I thought it would be worthwhile to give first a brief overview of the status of history of pharmacy courses in American schools of pharmacy.

A survey of the teaching of the history of pharmacy was recently completed by Robert A. Buerki of Ohio State University. Buerki surveyed all schools and colleges of pharmacy in the United States, Canada, Puerto Rico, and the Philippines.[1] His results indicate that of seventy-two schools in the United States (including one in Puerto Rico), twenty-eight (39 percent) offer a course in the history of pharmacy. Three of these institutions offer more than one course in the subject. Only seven of these schools (about 10 percent), however, require such a course. The great majority of the courses are offered on an elective basis.[2]

It is interesting to compare the results of the 1980–81 survey with those of the 1952 survey conducted by Glenn Sonnedecker and George Urdang.[3] In this earlier survey, thirty-six of the seventy schools of pharmacy, or slightly over 50 percent, offered a course in the history of pharmacy. Over the past three decades there has thus been a decline of about 20 percent in the number (and proportion) of pharmacy schools in which a history of pharmacy course is taught. When one compares the actual lists of the schools offering such courses in the two surveys, it is also apparent that there has been considerable turnover in the institutions involved.[4] The relatively large turnover suggests that whether or not a history course is offered at a given school may depend significantly upon local factors subject to change, such as the presence of an interested faculty member and/or a sympathetic dean.[5]

A striking figure from the 1952 survey is that twenty-eight of the thirty-six schools offering a course in the history of pharmacy reported that it was a part of the required curriculum.[6] As mentioned earlier, today there are only a handful of pharmacy schools that require such a course. Buerki has suggested that the pressure of other coursework, particularly in the clinical pharmacy area, has apparently been a significant factor in the trend toward eliminating the history of pharmacy course from the required curriculum.[7] It should be noted that some schools that do not require a history course would appear to incorporate some historical material into other courses, such as an orientation course.[8]

Most history of pharmacy courses are not taught by historians of pharmacy, but by interested faculty members from other disciplines within pharmacy (such as pharmaceutical chemistry) or by historians of science or medicine located elsewhere on the campus. It is fortunate that such individuals have developed an interest in the history of pharmacy, and their contributions to the field are invaluable. But I think there is a very real concern about the viability of the history of pharmacy as an academic discipline if there are too few trained historians devoting full time to the subject.[9]

The University of Wisconsin-Madison is recognized as the leading center for research and teaching in the history of pharmacy in this country. Wisconsin's School of Pharmacy has two historians on its staff, my colleague Glenn Sonnedecker and me. Madison is also the headquarters for the historical and publishing office of the American Institute of the History of Pharmacy, a national professional society of over a thousand members. Although the institute is independent of the university, the ties between the AIHP and Wisconsin's School of Pharmacy are very close. The AIHP director, for example, has always been a faculty member in Wisconsin's history of pharmacy program. Clearly the presence of the institute in Madison strengthens the academic program in history of pharmacy and vice versa.[10]

The tradition of teaching a course in the history of pharmacy goes back a long time at Wisconsin. Edward Kremers, who served as head of the pharmacy program from 1892 to 1935, introduced such a course in the first decade of this century.[11] In 1939, Kremers invited pharmacy historian George Urdang, a refugee from Nazi Germany, to Madison to collaborate on the writing of a textbook on the history of pharmacy.[12] The Kremers-Urdang book, now in its fourth edition as revised by Glenn Sonnedecker, has become the standard textbook and reference work in English on the subject.[13] Urdang remained in Madison after completion of the work, and in 1941 was the principal founder of the American Institute of the History of Pharmacy. Six years later he was made professor of the History of Pharmacy at Wisconsin, the first full-time professorship in the subject in the United States. In 1952, his student Glenn Sonnedecker became the first American to earn a Ph.D. in the history of pharmacy. Wisconsin remains the only American university to offer a doctorate specifically in pharmaceutical history. Its library resources in the history of pharmacy are clearly the best among American universities.

In light of this strong tradition of interest in pharmacy's past at

Wisconsin, it is not surprising that a course in the history of pharmacy is required of all pharmacy students. The school has felt that it is important for students to develop a perspective on their profession's heritage, and to be exposed to the humanistic dimensions of pharmacy. I might note that pharmacy students at Wisconsin are also required to take a course in "Social Aspects of American Pharmacy," taught by a sociologist on the faculty of the School of Pharmacy.[14]

The required history course is a three-credit course which covers the development of pharmacy in Western Europe and the United States from antiquity to the present, that is, a "survey" course. The emphasis is on the history of the pharmaceutical profession, with more limited attention given to the history of *materia medica* and drug therapy. About two-thirds of the course is devoted to the period since 1750, and about half of the course is devoted to pharmacy in the United States. Glenn Sonnedecker and I, who share the teaching of the course, have discussed on occasion whether it would be better to abandon the survey approach and limit the course to pharmacy since the Renaissance, or perhaps just to American pharmacy, since the average student's interest in a subject sometimes seems to diminish in direct proportion to the increase in time and distance from present-day America. We have continued to feel, however, that there is much value in tracing the roots of the profession back to ancient times. There is, of course, considerable room for disagreement about the relative advantages and disadvantages of the survey course versus a more limited and specialized course.

The basic structure and scope of the course may be outlined as follows:

1. Pharmacy's Early Antecedents (mainly 2000 B.C. to 1400 A.D.) (approximately 2 weeks)
   A. Primitive medicine and pharmacy
   B. Egypt and Mesopotamia
   C. Greece and Rome
   D. Emergence of pharmacy as a profession in the Middle Ages in Islam and Europe
2. Development of European Pharmacy (after 1400) (approximately 3 weeks)
   A. Renaissance innovations affecting pharmacy
   B. European pharmacist as scientist
   C. European pharmacist as practitioner
3. Pharmacy's Reflection in the Humanities (mainly since the seventeenth century, Europe and America) (approximately 1 week)
   A. Pharmacy in the literary and dramatic arts

      B. Pharmacy in music and the visual arts

      C. History of pharmacy, as a movement and as a hobby

4. Development of American Pharmacy (mainly after 1750) (approximately 6 weeks)

      A. American pharmacist as practitioner (pre-twentieth century)

      B. Legal controls related to pharmacy

      C. Pharmaceutical education

      D. The emergence of organized pharmacy

      E. American pharmacist as practitioner (twentieth century)

5. Trends Impacting upon Modern Pharmacy (mainly after 1800, Europe and America) (approximately 3 weeks)

      A. Changing concepts of disease

      B. Industrial Revolution and mass-produced medicines

      C. Modern science and technology

      D. Medicinal trademarks and patents

      E. "Third-party" methods of paying for medicines

      F. Growth of international cooperation

      G. The pharmacist in prospect

In the ancient period, since there was no identifiable profession of pharmacy, the emphasis is on the development of medical thought and the preparation and use of drugs. Attention is then focused on the emergence of pharmacy as a separate profession in the Middle Ages. The development of the profession is traced in selected European countries (Germany, France, Italy, Great Britain, and the Soviet Union), giving attention to similarities and differences in the evolution of pharmacy in diverse national contexts. We next turn to a very brief look at pharmacy's reflections in the humanities, particularly in the arts. Here, for example, we consider how the pharmacist has been portrayed in literature and visual art, the aesthetic aspects of the pharmacy and its equipment, the contributions to the arts by individual pharmacists, and the history of pharmacy itself as a discipline and as an avocational interest. Next, about six weeks are devoted to the development of pharmacy in the United States, including pharmaceutical legislation, education, and organization. Finally, the last three weeks of the course are devoted to forces and trends, both scientific-technological and social-economic, that have helped to shape modern pharmacy internationally. For example, we discuss the Industrial Revolution and the growth of a large-scale pharmaceutical manufacturing industry, the development of health insurance, and modern advances in drug therapy, considering in each case their impact on the profession of pharmacy.[15]

In addition to traditional lectures, we do make use of two other teaching techniques that I would like to discuss briefly, namely, the multimedia lecture and audio-tutorial methods. These methods were introduced in an effort to make the course more stimulating and meaningful to our large class (approximately 150 students). Student response to the methods has been good, and the general reaction to the course has also improved since these techniques were introduced.

The class meets three times a week, and one of these meetings each week is held in a special multimedia auditorium in the School of Education. This auditorium is equipped for rear-screen projection and allows for the use of slides (as many as five images may be projected simultaneously on the large screen), films, and video tapes. The room is also equipped with an overhead projector and a stereophonic sound system. Thus various media such as slides, films, and music may be integrated into the lecture in a programmed fashion. The push of a button by the lecturer may call up three slides onto the screen, or a slide accompanied by music, or a film or video tape. The multimedia approach has been in operation at Wisconsin since 1961, when Professor Michael Petrovich of the Department of History offered the first course utilizing this facility, a course on Russian history.

To date, Professor Sonnedecker and I have developed seven multimedia lectures, and it is our goal eventually to produce about fifteen, or one each week for the period that we meet in the multimedia auditorium. But the preparation of these lectures requires time and money, and hence our progress has not been as rapid as we might like.

We have also developed eight audio-tutorial units for use in the course. The audio-tutorial system may be less familiar to most historians, and to my knowledge it has received very little application in courses in the humanities, so I would like to discuss it in somewhat more detail. The audio-tutorial system of instruction involves the use of a variety of media to provide an integrated learning experience for the student on an independent study basis. The student goes to an audio-tutorial center (a room in the Pharmacy Library equipped with individual study carrels containing tape recorders, slide projectors, and various other materials) and is guided by a tutorial tape through a variety of activities. These may include showing slides, reading assigned materials, examining artifacts, and so on.

The audio-tutorial method was developed by Samuel N. Postlethwait of Purdue University in 1961 for his biology course.[17] Postlethwait's initial purpose was to provide supplementary lectures on tape which could be made available for the benefit of the weaker students in the class, but he soon observed that many students profited by listening to the tapes. He began to supplement the tapes with charts, photographs, slides, films, and other instructional aids, and eventually the taped lectures evolved into audio-tutorial units. In fact, students even carried out laboratory observations and experiments on their own with the guidance of the commentary on the tape.

We have adapted Postlethwait's method to our own purposes, although it has had to be significantly modified for use in history rather than biology or another science. Let me emphasize that these units are more than just slide-tape lectures. There is a certain amount of what we could call "lecturing" on the tapes, but the student does not simply sit back and listen to the tape and watch the slides flash by. We try, as much as possible, to get the student more actively involved in the learning process. The student may be asked to stop the tape and read an excerpt from the primary literature, and perhaps also to answer some question or questions concerning it. He may be asked to go to an exhibit case and examine the display there. Or he may be asked to examine an artifact placed at the audio-tutorial booth while the taped commentary points out certain features of it. He may be asked to show a slide and note some special point. In one unit the students listen to an excerpt from an interview that I conducted with a noted microbiologist who contributed to the development of large-scale penicillin manufacture.

There are a number of advantages to this type of instruction. For one thing, the student does become more actively involved in the learning process than in a lecture. The student also controls the unit. He shows the slides at his own pace, takes whatever time he feels is necessary for readings, goes over certain sections of the tape twice if he wishes, and so on. The information that the student receives on the subject is integrated into a single instructional unit. He is not reading an isolated excerpt from the Ebers Papyrus, for example, a day or a week after he has heard a lecture on Egyptian pharmacy. He reads the excerpt immediately after the taped commentary has explained the significance of the document and he has seen a slide of the Papyrus. The taped commentary also alerts him to points to watch for, or questions to ponder, as he reads the excerpt.

Although one might consider the method impersonal because it involves machines, it does allow for a certain kind of individualized instruction that would otherwise be impossible in a large class. The student can listen to the taped voice of an instructor commenting, for example, on an artifact that he holds in his hand, or a reading that is directly before him. He can examine a slide in detail at close range, rather than from the back of a lecture hall, and he can keep it on the screen as long as he wishes. The instructor can raise a question for the student to ponder, and have him stop the tape and develop his own answer before going on to hear what the instructor has to say on the subject. He can experience the unit at his convenience any time the library is open, and he controls the pace of the unit. We have found from experience that there may be as much as a 100 percent difference in the time spent on each unit by different students.

We would not wish to convert our whole course to the audio-tutorial approach, but have found it to be an effective supplement to other teaching methods; and the students have in general responded well to the technique. In weeks where an audio-tutorial unit is scheduled, one of the lectures is eliminated.

Because of the large number of students in the class and the lack of a teaching assistant for the course, we no longer conduct weekly discussion sections with small groups of students. We do schedule an optional review and question period before each of the three examinations, and encourage students to consult with us in our offices whenever they have questions or wish to discuss any subject with us. The textbook for the course is the previously mentioned *Kremers and Urdang's History of Pharmacy.*

I have presented a brief overview of the scope, content, and methods of the required history of pharmacy course at Wisconsin. Space does not permit detailed consideration of the elective course offerings, but I would like at least briefly to mention them as examples of the types of specialized elective courses that can be taught in the history of pharmacy area.[18]

A two-semester sequence on the history of drugs (either half of which may be taken independently) is regularly offered. The first-semester course covers the history of premodern *materia medica* and dosage forms (to about 1850) in relation to their natural origin and to the technology and science of processing by the pharmacist, with some attention also devoted to the rationale of therapeutic use. This course is aimed primarily at pharmacy students and includes laboratory exercises involving pharmaceutical botany and the compounding of traditional dosage forms. The second semester of the sequence treats the development of the major classes of modern therapeutic drugs (for example, biologicals, hormones, antibiotics) in relation to changing concepts of disease and drug action.

"Evolution of Food and Drug Controls" covers the historical development of standards and controls for foods and drugs, with emphasis on the United States in the nineteenth and twentieth centuries. "History of the Use and Misuse of Psychoactive Drugs" analyzes concepts, trends, and problems related to the use of psychoactive drugs throughout history. Both of these courses have drawn a significant proportion of their enrollment from outside the School of Pharmacy.

Finally, we will occasionally offer a seminar devoted to a specific theme in the history of pharmacy or the pharmaceutical sciences: for example, the history of pharmacology.

It seems clear that the role of a historian in a professional school must go beyond teaching and research in the history of the subject. I believe that the historian should serve also as a representative of the liberal arts tradition and encourage the inclusion of courses in the humanities and social sciences in the overall program of the professional student. A course in the history of the student's intended profession can serve as an important part of a program designed to expose him to humanistic, ethical, and social concerns, but cannot in itself completely fulfill these goals.[19]

Notes

1. Robert A. Buerki, "History of pharmacy courses in schools and colleges of pharmacy: preliminary results of a survey" (Paper delivered at the Workshop on Teaching the History of Pharmacy, Annual Meeting of the American Institute of the History of Pharmacy, St. Louis, 30 March 1981). *Amer. J. Pharm. Ed.,* in press.

2. In the version of this paper delivered at the conference in October 1980, the results I presented were based on an earlier (1976) and less complete survey by Professor Buerki, and hence differed slightly from the figures presented here (taken from n. 1 above). See Robert A. Buerki, "Teaching the history of pharmacy: a preliminary assessment," *Teaching the History and Sociology of Pharmacy* (newsletter issued by the American Institute of the History of Pharmacy, Madison, Wis.), No. 1, May 1977, pp 1–3.

3. Glenn Sonnedecker and George Urdang, "A survey of the status of history of pharmacy in American pharmaceutical education," *Amer. J. Pharm. Ed.,* 1952, *16:* 11–21.

4. This relatively high turnover can be confirmed by comparing the list of schools that taught history of pharmacy courses in 1952 and in 1981. The 1952 report only identified the schools that required a history of pharmacy course, but since those schools constituted 78 percent (28 of 36) of the institutions offering such a course, this list may be used for the purposes of making a rough comparison. Only six colleges appear on both lists. Although this figure is no doubt somewhat low due to the incompleteness of the 1952 list, it is still obvious that there has been considerable turnover.

5. For example, in the 1976 survey nine schools listed lack of qualified teaching personnel as a reason for decreased emphasis or discontinued coursework in history of pharmacy. Buerki, "Teaching the history of pharmacy," p. 2. Five of the respondents to the 1981 survey indicated that the death or retirement of a faculty member led to the elimination of a history of pharmacy course. Buerki, "History of pharmacy courses," p. 4

6. Sonnedecker and Urdang, "Survey," pp. 14–15.

7. Buerki, "History of pharmacy courses," p. 4. In 1976, seventeen schools listed increased emphasis on clinical coursework as a reason for decreased emphasis or discontinued coursework in history of pharmacy. Buerki, "Teaching the history of pharmacy," pp. 2–3.

8. Professor Buerki has also compiled data on such courses. See Buerki, "History of pharmacy courses," pp. 4–6.

9. The University of Wisconsin may be the only American school of pharmacy that has on its faculty trained historians devoting full time to the history of pharmacy.

10. On the founding and history of the first twenty years of the institute's existence, see Ernst Stieb, *American Institute of the History of Pharmacy: Through Two Decades* (Madison, Wis.: American Institute of the History of Pharmacy, 1961).

11. On Kremers, see George Urdang, "Edward Kremers (1865–1941): reformer of American pharmaceutical education," *Amer. J. Pharm. Ed.,* 1947, *11:* 631–58.

12. On Urdang, see H. George Wolfe, "George Urdang, 1882–1960: the man and his work," *Pharmacy in History,* 1960, *5:* 33–42.

13. Edward Kremers and George Urdang, *History of Pharmacy: A Guide and a Survey* (Philadelphia: J. B. Lippincott, 1940). The latest edition is *Kremers and Urdang's History of Pharmacy,* 4th ed. rev. (Philadelphia: J. B. Lippincott, 1976).

14. Associate Professor Bonnie Svarstad. The School of Pharmacy offers graduate degrees in pharmaceutical sociology as well as pharmaceutical history.

15. A copy of the course syllabus may be obtained from the author upon request.

16. For further information on the multimedia instructional facilities at Wisconsin, contact the Instructional Media-Distribution Center, 142 Educational Sciences Building, University of Wisconsin, Madison, Wis. 53706.

17. S. N. Postlethwait, J. Novak, and H. T. Murray, Jr., *The Audio-Tutorial Approach to Learning through Independent Study and Integrated Experiences*, 2d ed. (Minneapolis: Burgess, 1969).

18. Syllabi of any of the courses mentioned below may be obtained from the author upon request.

19. For a recent discussion of liberal arts in the pharmacy curriculum, see David A. Fedo, "Liberal arts and pharmacy education: where do we now stand?," *Pharmacy in History*, 1980, *22:* 60–68.

COMMENTARY—CINDERELLA AND BIG SISTER: A CASE FOR CLOSER RELATIONSHIPS

J. K. Crellin

Historians of medicine sometimes play the role of the mean step-sister and look upon the history of pharmacy as a Cinderella. Their indifference to the benefits of pharmaceutical perspectives on certain medical issues often leads to gaps in scholarship. I am pleased, therefore, to be given the opportunity to comment on John Parascandola's essay and also, as I have been asked, to raise questions about the history of medicine in a medical center and the part the history of pharmacy might play.

I. John Parascandola has spoken of more than forty years of sustained research and teaching of the history of pharmacy at the University of Wisconsin-Madison. Together with the American Institute of the History of Pharmacy, they have made singular contributions to the profession of pharmacy. I think that it is appropriate to add that, in its activities, the institute has been more attentive to the needs of its individual members than the American Association for the History of Medicine, though I hasten to add that this is not a criticism of the AAHM as much as a reflection on the good fortune of AIHP in having a permanent location and long-serving directors. Yet, despite Parascandola's Wisconsin success story, he has, in documenting a recent decline in the number of pharmacy schools teaching the history of pharmacy, provided a dismal picture. In so doing Parascandola enters territory familiar to historians of medicine; namely, failure to have a major impact on a profession as a whole, be it medicine or pharmacy.

It can, of course, be argued that our task as historians of medicine is to cater only to those who come to us fully committed to the subject, and that our major concern should be to spend a large part of our time on research, writing, and publishing. The latter activities are essential, but the tenor of the times, as some of the other contributors have already indicated, is against full-time commitment, or, for that matter, waiting in the wings for students to appear. In recent years, this has been recognized by many determined efforts to make history of medicine courses more popular. Stressing aspects of the history of medicine that seem to have special relevance to medicine today and ensuring that attention is paid to the social context amid which medicine changes, with the idea of improving the general intellectual value of a course, are two ways of doing this. Both those areas have a conspicuous part in the discussions in this symposium and I am very supportive of them. I believe firmly that we have to be watchful of the demands of the marketplace. We must make a contribution to the general medical scene in a medical center, not only by providing sustenance to those interested in history, but also by stimulating nonhistory "buffs" to think just a little more critically of the enterprise of medicine as a whole.

In order to make history of medicine as relevant and as intellectually stimulating as possible, historians of medicine might profitably look to history of pharmacy for appropriate material. For instance, topics on the history of therapy (for example, pharmacists' contributions to dosage forms) can be helpful in providing perspectives on such current issues as patients' compliance in taking prescribed medicines, whereas consideration of changing attitudes of pharmacists to physicians as well as the recent "clinical pharmacy" movement can help illuminate some of the stresses and strains of twentieth-century medicine.

I could at this juncture list many other areas of the history of pharmacy that would be of interest to medical students and then go on to discuss some situations that many of us would consider ideal. For instance, a situation where medical students, pharmacy students, and students in other health fields would join together for interdisciplinary courses on the history of the health professions. However, I doubt if this course could be applied generally. Time constraints will always limit the number of examples from history of pharmacy that can be included in history of medicine courses (though, of course, not medical history research) and, in the current climate, it is unlikely that more than a handful of centers will be able to organize courses for interdisciplinary audiences, unless the optimism for the growth of "medical humanities" is justified.

II. I prefer to devote the rest of my comment to a totally different issue, one that I believe all centers might find relevant and that allows a different consideration of my theme of relationships between history of pharmacy and history of medicine. In pondering over the failure of history of medicine to achieve a greater impact than it has in recent years, and in reflecting on such current concerns as the disappearance of the amateur historian, I begin to wonder whether historians of medicine have concentrated too much attention on education within the formal classroom setting. One wonders if more attention should have been paid to making medical centers regional centers for history of medicine.

Should a center with a history of medicine program generate activity in the hope of creating a good level of interest in a region, which might result in a healthy groundswell of support for that center? To some extent, of course, we are all involved in at least sending out ripples of history of medicine, if only through responding to invitations to address a variety of audiences. At Duke, if I can refer to my current experience, we have sponsored more than just ad hoc activities by individuals—for example, a conference on local history and a course on medical botany, the latter ostensibly for those associated with the North Carolina Botanical Gardens. These evoked encouraging responses and led to the creation of a regular newsletter called "Medicine in North Carolina." Thoughts are now being directed toward a systematic program of generating activity in a region.

Such a program can include, for example: regular conferences; lecture courses; newsletters and publications; the preparation of slide talks for laymen (e.g., changes in infant feeding practices, the growth of drug addiction, and the industrial archeology of medicine); the preparation of exhibitions for use within and outside a medical center; and the use of local museums for teaching purposes. The latter can be useful in expanding the variety of presentations for medical students and can provide another way of incorporating history of pharmacy. We at Duke are fortunate in having four museums with sizable medical and pharmaceutical collections within manageable driving distances for half-day sessions. All have pharmacies providing us with an appropriate environment, in which to discuss with students, the story of medicine and pharmacy for the eighteenth century, the late nineteenth century, and the 1920s and 1930s. Two of the museums also have doctors' offices representative of the late nineteenth century. The museums allow historians—in a relatively short time—to weave pictures of the daily life of a physician who dispensed his own medicines, as well as to study the development of diagnostic instruments and therapy. In turn, those topics readily raise questions about the growing professional identity of pharmacy in the nineteenth century, encouraging a symbiosis of facets from the two disciplines of the history of medicine and history of pharmacy, without extending teaching time.

The museum curators with whom we have dealt invariably welcome any use of their facilities for teaching purposes, if only because this helps them develop fresh insights into their collections. In that manner curators can readily become very much part of a medical center's regional activities.

III. I have suggested that the quest for producing a greater impact from medical history programs should include regional roles apart from the traditional ones of contributing to scholarship and teaching within a classroom setting. In so doing I believe that we can enlarge our intellectual service to the medical profession, and, in return, history programs in medical centers will receive much benefit. I hope, too, that I have given some ideas where history of pharmacy might profitably be used to elucidate facets of the history of medicine without being unrealistic by suggesting new or extended courses.

In concluding, I would like to say some words about my title Cinderella (history of pharmacy) and Big Sister (history of medicine). I have indicated that they have common problems, although I have restricted my remarks to Big Sister, the theme of this symposium, suggesting she should not be so aloof—at least to some aspects of the history of pharmacy. But what about Cinderella's problems? Why is the history of pharmacy losing ground, particularly in a time when there is considerable emphasis placed on liberal education? Maybe, and I am saying this in a constructive rather than critical spirit, the history of pharmacy is not paying sufficient attention to its own marketplace. At a time when much of pharmacy education—through the thrust of "clinical pharmacy"—is trying to give students a better appreciation of the dynamics of medicine, particularly in the area of physician-patient relationships, should not historians of pharmacy be incorporating more history of medicine—or at least selected aspects—into their courses? I think the evidence many of us have gained in teaching allied health students shows how receptive such students generally are to the history of medicine, particularly when topics are considered that highlight the stresses and strains of twentieth-century medicine. Perhaps, in a perverse sort of way, pharmacy students would be more receptive to the history of medicine than the history of pharmacy. If survey courses are to persist—and that question was raised by John Parascandola—could not more room be found for relevant history of medicine. I am convinced Cinderella and Big Sister could profitably improve their relationships for the mutual benefit of each other. Unhappily, there is no Prince Charming. We all have to contribute in terms of deeds rather than words if there is to be a happy ending.

THE HISTORY OF MEDICINE IN A MEDICAL CONTEXT

Pauline M. H. Mazumdar

I propose to discuss the relation of the history of medicine to the life experience of the student audience: both the social context in which the students live, and the intellectual context of their medical thought.

Let me start by saying something about my own experiences. We began our history of medicine program at the University of Toronto in 1977, so it is a relatively recent addition to the teaching there. This is a university with undergraduate teaching, a strong graduate school, and a number of professional schools such as medicine, pharmacy, and engineering. The program we offer in the history of medicine is a three-tier one: an undergraduate survey course, which is offered also as an elective to the medical students; a graduate seminar, which is part of the Master's program in the history of science; and a research seminar for people who have been through this teaching program and are at the Ph.D. level. The part of the program I shall address myself to is the part with the problem: that is, the undergraduate-*cum*-medical students lectures. It is a survey course of twenty-two two-hour lectures, with some reading each week, an hour's tutorial in smaller groups and an examination and research paper. The current course description reads:

> The theme of these lectures is the intimate relationship of medicine with the history and culture of its time. Medical theories and practices of the past and the social pressures which moulded them will be discussed and illustrated wherever possible with contemporary visual material—instruments, vase paintings, mediaeval manuscript illustrations, cartoons and photographs.

We offer this as a voluntary elective with no written requirements—either examination or paper—for the medical students, and as an ordinary college course to the undergraduates. Figure 1 shows how the student audiences have turned out in the course's first three years.[1]

The first year (1977–78) was on a small scale; I tried out the seminar form with a few medical students. It was not very successful; the medical students did not have time to do enough reading to sustain a small group seminar. Furthermore, their approach to discussion of the

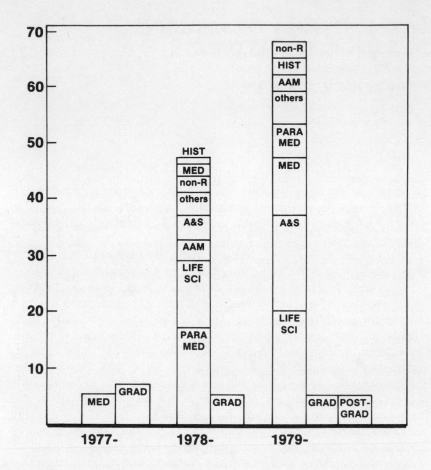

FIGURE 1. History of Medicine 1977–78, 1978–79, 1979–80 Student Audience Analysis.

PARA-MED: physiotherapy, occupational therapy, nursing, health sciences, pharmacy, massage, speech pathology

LIFE SCI: anatomy, physiology, zoology, psychology, biology, biochemistry, microbiology, pre-med and pre-dental

MED: 1st, 2nd and 3rd yr. medical students on elective

AAM: students from Faculty of Art as Applied to Medicine

others: including philosophy, commerce, 'special' students

non-R: unregistered auditors including hospital residents, faculty members, etc.

HIST: history and history of science

GRAD and POST-GRAD: students mainly in M.A. and Ph.D. history of science

A&S: Arts and Sciences; students who have not yet specialized material was not critical enough: they tried to learn it, rather than to criticize it. So the following year (1978–79) we put on a lecture course instead, and opened it to undergraduates as well. The audience for the 1979–80 consisted of these groups:

25% Life sciences
25% Arts and sciences
25% Miscellaneous
15% Paramedical
10% Medical students

Only 10 percent of our 1979 student audience were actual medical students on voluntary electives—and many of them did not attend regularly. The medical students receive no official credit for electives, so there is no pressure here for them to excel as there would be in their core classes. There is insufficient intellectual payoff in it to make up for that, except in the case of the exceptional individual, of whom we have had a few. History of medicine is just not one of the tools they all need to learn their trade. Both the students and the curriculum committee recognize that.

This has not always been the case. In the past, historians of medicine could claim that their work had a practical payoff; it could be used to help the student understand the reasons for choosing one type of medical theory rather than another. I am thinking in this regard of Daniel Leclerc's book of 1696. Its title, *Histoire de la médecine ou l'on void l'origine et le progrès de cet art de siècle en siècle depuis le commencemen du monde,* reads rather like a modern survey course. The preface declares his purpose; a certain Dr. Lionardo di Capoa has written a history of medicine which aims to show how useless all traditional medical systems have been, and how only modern medicine, founded on physics and chemistry—eighteenth-century iatromechanics and iatrochemistry, of course—are any good. Leclerc accuses this writer of stepping out of his role as historian by using that position to refute sentiments which are not to his taste. The principal use of this book, says Leclerc, is to open the eyes of those who are too respectful of the ancients; but, he points out, no one has ever yet written a properly *balanced* history of medicine. Doctors usually write books that tend to show at its best everything coinciding with their own opinion; what Leclerc will do is try to enter into the spirit of every age, of each author, and report faithfully what belongs to each. That is true history, he says. But here he shows his hand at last, for his appointed task will be to give to the ancients what is theirs and not ascribe to the moderns what does not belong to them:

One discovers, among the fables of Aesculapius and other divine physi-

cians, traces of the remedies which we still use today almost everywhere, as
the mainstays of medicine—such as bleeding and purging, whose antiquity
is thus established.[2]

And there you have his position: Leclerc is using his history of medicine
as a means of combating the new iatromechanics and iatrophysics. In
the battle of the books, Leclerc is for the ancients rather than the
moderns. For the students, this controversy would have had direct
relevance; it would be part of their choice of tools for the trade, and
immediately relevant in their life experience.

One can imagine Boerhaave including Lionardo di Capoa's history,
and not Daniel Leclerc's, among the books he recommended to his
students to read in his *Method of Studying Physic* (1719). He tells them:

> Now all those who wrote before the year 1628 whether *Greeks* or *Latins,*
> are good for nothing; for they were Strangers to the Harvean System of the
> Circulation of the Blood. For this is the only principal Cause on which
> depends all the rest: For what signifies it that we know the structure of the
> parts, unless we know by what Order Force and Velocity the Humours con-
> tinually flow throughout them? But this before the Year 1628 was
> altogether unknown.[3]

And he goes on to tell the students that in advising them what to read,
one must act with great prudence, and speak of none but those that will
be worth their while to study; that is, those who lay down no principles
except those of physics and chemistry.

Both Leclerc's and Lionardo di Capoa's histories are relevant for the
student's practical learning of medicine: Leclerc who points out for
them the reliability of the old therapy, purging and bloodletting; and
Lionardo who explains to them the new theory and its origins. They
need to know both, and the historians are able to provide what they
need. The history of medicine at this time and for long afterwards was
pragmatic—as Kurt Sprengel put it in 1821. He called his history in fact,
Versuch einer pragmatischen Geschichte der Arzneykunde.

> A history is pragmatic when it makes us wiser . . . letting us better under-
> stand the structure of medical thought: it shows us the use of even wrong
> attempts to understand the truth and helps towards the improvement of our
> own system of medicine.[4]

His contemporary Emile Littré, in translating Hippocrates into French,
had the same point of view in 1839:

> My purpose has been to put the Hippocratic works completely at the
> disposal of the physicians of our time: I have hoped that they might be read
> and understood like a contemporary work.[5]

And he says in his preface, "When antique and modern thought make
contact thus, they *fecundate* each other"; it is an image which suggests

the intimately intense relationship that Littré imagined between his contemporary and the physician of antiquity.[6] Hippocrates may have
lacked a knowledge of modern pathology—the localization of diseases
in organs—but he knew about the general disease state. Although Hippocratic medicine had its lacunae, for Littré it formed a solid base for
contemporary medicine; it gave the physician of 1840 an understanding
of the states common to all kinds of disease, as well as of the influence
of climate on constitution. To this Littré's contemporaries have added a
knowledge of species of disease; but he thinks that the earlier
knowledge is as valid as ever.

Even in 1860, a history of medicine could still be used to present a
choice between two types of doctrine; Wunderlich's history is still
history as written—like Daniel Leclerc's of 1696—to present a particular point of view within medicine, rather than within historiography.
Wunderlich's organizing principle is the conflict between the physiological and the ontological viewpoints: he presents himself as the
founder of nineteenth-century physiological medicine, which has swept
away the Paracelsian ontology of an earlier time. Wunderlich and his
new physiological medicine are the natural goal of history to which it
has all been tending.

> The expression "physiological medicine" which we chose was intended to
> express our rejection of all ontological and personificatory concepts in
> pathology: pathology is only the physiology of the sick man; it also served
> to remind us that the same methods and means for the ascertainment of
> facts, the same kind of logic were needed as in the science of the healthy
> body. This expression became the slogan of the age and many people
> boasted that they belonged to this school of thought even though they had
> neither understood the problem nor had the means to practice the
> methods.[7]

They should learn to handle the new tools, he is telling them; his new
tool for physiological medicine was the thermometer. This tool is
within the life experience of the practicing physician or student. It is
something which involves the physician's bedside procedure.

The present position of the history of medicine is that it is no longer
involved in the physician's choice of action: the historian of medicine is
no longer an advocate speaking from within the profession, using
history in an attempt to guide his students along some particular professional path—telling them, as it were, that history is on our side. It has
not done this now at least since Edelstein suggested that the Hippocratic
oath was not an ethical ideal for all physicians of all times, but the oath
of a Pythagorean sect, relevant not to us now, but to the sectarian then.[8]

But we are, at that point, still within the realm of the history of
ideas: and so far the professional student can follow us. This is the style
that present-day good professional students generally adopt when

writing about the history of medicine. Here, for example, is a citation from a paper written by Sandra Black when she was one of our medical students: this essay won the Osler Prize last year. Dr. Black is writing about theories of the transmission of nerve impulses across a synapse:

> In a long review of neuron theory published in 1893, Tanzi proposed that the passage of impulses between neurons produced a "functional hypertrophy" of the transmitting neurons which was comparable to the hypertrophy of muscle fibres with exercise . . . the distance between the neurons at the interneural junctions was correspondingly decreased . . . conduction was inversely related to the size of the functional gap and therefore . . . 'exercise' facilitated future conduction over that junction by decreasing the interneuronal distance.[9]

This essay has had a lot of praise—justly, I think. It is very good of its kind, and it discusses the ideas that are the antecedents of the ideas that Dr. Black herself uses: she is a resident in neurology now. It discusses them with great analytical insight, but without any suggestion that the neurologists of 1890 were people in a real world, with real conditions and constraints to thought. But even this student is not an ordinary medical student: she spent some time working with Charles Webster in Oxford. We have two other outstanding individuals involved in medicine who may produce comparable work, and like Dr. Black they are not ordinary medical students: one is a graduate student in physiology and one in experimental surgery, and they take part in our graduate seminars.

So we are left with the position that history of medicine is no longer pragmatic enough to be *needed* by the ordinary medical student. The exceptional individuals—mainly people of great talent on the edge of the profession—will continue to respond and to produce good work. I expect that it will mostly be something like Dr. Black's in style—the style of history of ideas.

The mainstream of history, however—that is, the history issuing from history departments—is no longer the history of ideas. Figure 2 was constructed by Robert Darnton of Princeton for his essay on "Intellectual and cultural history," which appeared in a recent group of essays on American historiography.[10]

The implication is plain to see. In American universities, courses in intellectual history are about as numerous as those in social history, and publications in the two fields are about the same as well; this represents the work of our generation. But Ph.D. dissertations in social history now enormously outnumber those in intellectual history, pointing to a coming growth in social history in the next generation. As historians of medicine we should take pretty seriously what the history departments are doing. Their relation to us is a bit like that of the United States to Canada: bigger, and *very* influential. And, I imagine, what is happening

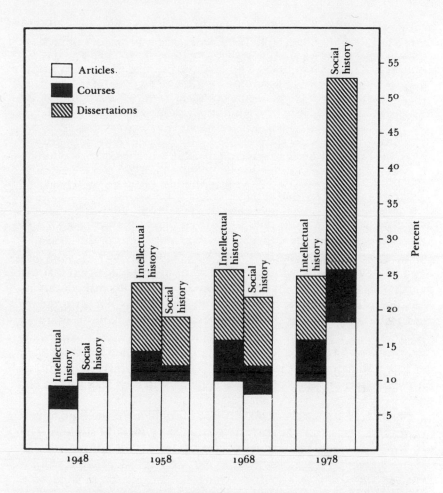

FIGURE 2. Articles, Courses, and Dissertations in Intellectual and Social History as Percentages of All History Articles, Courses, and Dissertations. Reprinted by permission from Robert Darnton, "Intellectual and cultural history" in Michael Kammen, *The Past before Us: Contemporary Historical Writing in the United States* (Ithaca, N.Y.: Cornell University Press, 1980), p. 336.

to them is what will soon be happening to the history of medicine. It is doing so already.

So what are we left with as teachers of the history of medicine in a medical center? Our medical students probably want something that no historian can now give them: pragmatic history. Our exceptional individuals within the profession will stick to the history of ideas; the ideas are, after all, their own. What then will happen to our audience as more and more of us move into social history, or at least begin to deal with the social referents of medicine?

I suggest that we do what our Toronto student audience is indicating: that we teach history of medicine to the students who are not yet personally involved with the profession, but who are interested in it as outsiders. These are students who do have the time to invest in a heavy course with a lot of reading: who are prepared to put a lot into it, and therefore get a lot out. They will then be entering medicine as a profession *after* having done a year's course in its history. They will become aware of the social moulding of the profession and of medical thought *before* they become involved in the profession themselves. These people may acquire and retain a historical orientation which may then persist through their professional training, and even through their absorption into the professional ethos.

The new policy I am proposing is to conform officially to what the figures tell us has been happening. We should retain the electives, but we should encourage undergraduates in the university who want to apply to the medical school to take the history of medicine course. In this way a much larger proportion of medical students will in fact have taken the course than happens now. They will be taking it far more seriously too, not simply as auditors but as regular full-load students. We hope that this indirect approach to the problem will be more successful than the direct one has been: we will not be teaching the history of medicine to the medical profession, but the medical profession will in fact have been taught it. Perhaps in this way we will be able to reconcile the needs of the historians with the needs of their audience.

Notes

1. P. M. H. Mazumdar, *Report for the Review Committee,* Jason A. Hannah Chair in History of Medicine, November 1979, Appendix I.

2. Daniel Leclerc, in the "Avertissement" to *Histoire de la médecine, ou l'on void l'origine et les progrés de cet art, de siécle en siécle depuis le commencemen du monde* (Amsterdam, 1723).

3. H. Boerhaave, *A Method of Studying Physick,* trans. Samber (London: Rivington, 1719), p. 254.

4. Kurt Sprengel, *Versuch einer pragmatischen Geschichte der Arzneykunde,* 6 vols. (Halle: Gebauer, 1821–1840), 1:4.

5. Emile Littré, ed. and trans., *Oeuvres completes d'Hippocrate,* 2 vols. (Paris: Balliere, 1839), 1:ix.

6. Littré, *Ibid.,* 1:xiv.

7. C. A. Wunderlich, *Geschichte der Medizin* (Stuttgart: Ebner, 1859), p. 357.

8. L. Edelstein, "The Hippocratic oath: text, translation, and interpretation," in *Ancient Medicine: Selected Papers of Ludwig Edelstein* (Baltimore: The Johns Hopkins Press, 1967), pp. 3–64.

9. S. Black, "Pseudopods and synapses: the amoeboid theories of neuronal mobility and the early formulation of the synapse concept, 1894–1900," *Bull. Hist. Med.,* 1981, 5: 34–58.

10. Robert Darnton, "Intellectual and cultural history," in M. Kammen, *The Past before Us: Contemporary Historical Writing in the United States* (Ithaca, N.Y.: Cornell University Press, 1980), p. 336.

COMMENTARY: IS NONINTELLECTUALISM INVADING THE MEDICAL SCHOOL?*

Edward C. Atwater

Not long ago I became interested in the mottos of colleges and universities. My curiosity, and the help of a Latin-literate colleague, led me to a three-category classification. An approximate translation is provided for those who wish it.

First are those expressing religious belief: Brown's "In Deo speramus" (Our hope is in God), Wooster's "Ex uno fonte" (From one source), or Princeton's "Dei sub numine viget" (It flourishes by the presence of God).

The largest group is of the light-truth-peace-freedom-knowledge type: Tufts's "Pax et lux," Yale's "Lux et veritas," Harvard's "Veritas," Columbia's "In litteris libertas" (In education is liberty), Syracuse's "Suos cultores scientia coronat" (Knowledge crowns those who cultivate it), Rochester's "Meliora" (Better things), and Amherst's "Terras irradient" (Let them illuminate the earth). Note that these come from Massachusetts, Connecticut, and New York.

Then there are the ethical or moral types, which seem to come from Pennsylvania and Vermont: Pennsylvania's "Leges sine moribus vanae" (Law without morality is useless), Vermont's "Studiis et rebus honestis" (By study and honest dealing), or Middlebury's "Scientia et virtute" (By knowledge and virture).

Some schools no longer make much use of their seals and mottos, and perhaps this is significant since often the words seem inappropriate to the fact. Certainly faith in God is largely gone, and it is often difficult to perceive the search for light and truth amid the present public relations bombardment in the press. This is especially the case in medical schools. There, nonintellectualism seems to have been on the increase during the past thirty years.

Only a few mottos seem adaptable to current needs. Perhaps City College of New York's "Respice, adspice, prospice" could be interpreted "Keep your eyes open, they may be gaining on you." Or that of the Medical College of Pennsylvania—"Droit et avant"—might be

*Dr. Mazumdar's paper was not yet available when these remarks were prepared.

"Right on!" in contemporary idiom. Dartmouth's motto, "Vox clamantis in deserto," speaks well of the plight of a nonscience scholar in the medical center. So does the University of Salamanca's motto. Dr. Jarcho recalls, but does not vouch, that it said: "What God has not given, this University will not provide."

Is there evidence for nonintellectualism? I recently attended an AOA lecture—it was open to the general public—and was intrigued by the fact that the speaker, a surgeon, could give such a scholarly and entertaining talk on the literature of surgery. My enthusiasm was later dampened while discussing it with a colleague. I heard what for many is the ultimate judgment of any report today: "Yes, it was good but he could not get a grant."

Not long after this I overheard a medical student complaining about the time he was obliged to waste in physiology laboratory, repeating experiments that had once, long ago, led to some new knowledge. "Why not just stay home and read the book." As he saw it, he would save time, be more certain of understanding the point, and surer of passing the exam.

At an even earlier level of undifferentiation is the premed, forty thousand of whom struggle each year for one of the seventeen thousand places in American medical schools. Faced with legal prerequisites in chemistry, biology, and physics, with MCAT tests, and with admissions committees usually dominated by laboratory scientists, to say nothing of the ambitious parent who always wanted a physician in the family, there is little time for academic pursuits that may seem then peripheral to the goal. Scientific literacy will make the applicant victorious in the engagement at hand, though inability to express himself in English will become all too apparent when he enters the clinical years and must record patient histories and contribute to medical journals.

Now more than ever before, children at the earliest stage of intellectual curiosity are being overwhelmed with communications from many sources—the media—especially television and radio. They are never alone, it is never quiet, but, no matter, there is no need to read—either for information or for company. There develops little desire to seek out, to discover. Though conditioned to compete and succeed, many become intellectually passive.

In order to assess the general medical knowledge of young physicians, a simple quiz in which the student was asked to associate thirty-four famous names in medicine with thirty-four phrases, one of which was associated with each of the names (for example, Fleming and penicillin), was given to medical students. The results: among sixty-eight third-year medical students the mean number of names correctly identified was twelve or 35 percent. Later the same quiz was taken by twenty-four medical residents who did only slightly better. Fifteen RIs and RIIs had a mean of fifteen correct and nine RIIIs had a mean of seventeen. Both the students and residents did best on names associated with genetics and radiology. No student was able to associate Enders with growing viruses in vitro or Auenbrugger with percussion. Only one associated Hippocrates with Cos, and five or less appropriately identified Bernard, Semmelweis, Liebig, Beaumont, Sims, or Pierre Louis. Only with Beaumont, Bernard, and Sims were the residents slightly better. Only five of thirty-four residents associated the stethoscope with Laennec. Less than half the students associated Lister with antisepsis, Vesalius with human anatomy, Jenner with cowpox, Pasteur with disproving spontaneous generation, Banting with insulin, or Koch with tubercle bacillus.

I do not suggest that these data by themselves are solid proof of anti- or nonintellectualism, but I do believe that such a lack of general knowledge among those who represent some of our brightest youth, compounded with some of the attitudes and behavior I mentioned, do reflect narrow interests.

Nor do I propose that all of this is new. Situations similar to these have always existed. But I think the condition is more prevalent in recent decades. The student as well as the physician is pressed today by external demands that he or she work toward a finite goal and present a product; and success is measured in productivity. Even patient care has been replaced by a product called "health care," which is distributed and delivered to consumers. Physicians are addressed by the bureaucracy as "Dear Provider," a fact that betrays a fundamental misconception of what a physician is or should be.

This is the heart of the problem. Medicine has become more dependent on objective evaluations and impersonal procedures and less dependent on relationships between people. This, in itself, is not necessarily bad, but it has led, inevitably, to a loss of care while the product has improved and that *is* bad.

The brilliance of some of these procedures is distracting. It is hard to resist the tempting idea that if research has led to these innovations then we should concentrate all of our energy on achieving more of these successes and forget the rest, overlooking or ignoring that vast body of problems which still resists technological solution. If physicians fail to develop nonscientific attributes, as well, they will be giving up the tradition of 2,000 years, replacing a learned profession with a cadre of sophisticated technicians.

This issue is heavily influenced by how we pay for medical education and for medical care. If medical education continues to receive (as it does) more than half of its financial support from the taxpayer, through government grants, and if the reward system for patient care continues to be so heavily skewed toward procedures, it will be difficult to encourage breadth. Individual taxpayers and the industries that support the insurance system are understandably disinterested in intellectual things; they want tangible results for their money, results that can be defined and tabulated. In such an atmosphere, interest in pursuits such as philosophy or language or history will not thrive. It is not hard to understand then why historical pursuits do not engender much interest among physicians these days, nor even among medical faculties and the students who learn to copy them as children do their parents.

The premed will not believe that prowess in English or philosophy or history, with limited though substantial scientific attainments, is likely to lead to an offer of a place in medical school. With exceptions, he is correct in his perception. The humanities major almost inevitably has difficulty in the first two years of medical school and the admissions committee is called upon to justify having risked even one slot on such a person. Even students admitted to medical school at the end of their sophomore year in college, with the specific intention of relieving them of the premed pressure, and who are thus encouraged to broaden their education, almost invariably accelerate their science track. So it cannot all be blamed on premed pressure.

The medical student in physiology has little interest in the historical continuum, the process of discovery, and where the sequence of events might likely lead. His goal is more immediate—to pass the exam. The professor, a bit older, rather likes the idea of medical history (but is frequently embarrassed to say so) but success, even survival, means grants and that means data and papers that peers with similar motivation think will lead to other advances.

Until a simpler way of life returns, and it seems unlikely that it will, or until a less goal-oriented physician is being produced, or perhaps until substantial extramural support becomes available to medical faculties for teaching and scholarship in the humanities, the situation will not change much. The internally competitive and goal-oriented student who matriculates in American medical schools, and who, once there, is looked upon favorably by faculty and peers, cannot afford the diverting luxury of much intellectual curiosity that is peripheral to the secrets of biological science.

OCCUPYING THE VISUAL CORTEX: USING SLIDES TO TEACH THE HISTORY OF MEDICINE*

Robert J. T. Joy

Professional historians of medicine are continually exploring ways to teach or better teach the history of medicine to men and women who have chosen one of the health professions as a career. My experience is limited to teaching medical students, house officers, and nurses, and giving medical history talks to physicians in continuing medical education programs. While I believe these suggestions will be useful in teaching undergraduates or students in other health professions, I cannot speak from experience.

Our students grew up with television. They have been conditioned to learn by an audio-visual technology. It has been estimated that they have already done twenty thousand hours of TV watching, or have spent more time before a TV set than in class.[1] While they are our students, they continue to watch television. Educational psychologists report that on the average 75 percent of learning is done visually; only 25 percent of our stored data enter through our ears.[2] This paper suggests a method of exploiting these two facts, and of using our students' eyes to help teach them the history of medicine.

In spite of the myriad experiments with computer-assisted education, with the use of film or video tape, with seminars, workshops, and laboratory conference teaching, it remains true that the lecture is and will remain the basic teaching method. It is traditional, efficient for large groups, reasonably effective, inexpensive, and—most importantly—puts a living person in the arena who can answer questions, respond to audience mood and affect, and communicate a sense of personal investment in the subject. What I propose here is an addition to and reinforcement for the standard lecture—the use of large numbers of 2 x 2 slides to accompany the lecture.

If one accepts as a given that cortical arousal is increased by added stimulation and that information is more likely to be attended to and retained, then adding pictures to words will improve nearly any lecture.[3] Many teachers of the history of medicine use slides—most do

*A more informal version of this paper, accompanied by eighty slides, was presented at the conference.

not. Many of those who do, use only a few slides in the usual fifty-minute lecture, or have not considered the variety of ways in which historical information can be displayed with slides. I suggest here several tactics that may be helpful to those who use pictorial material, and I hope to arouse an interest in their use by those who do not.

Most of our students have not had much education in history beyond a high school or college survey course. They usually remember a random collection of "important" events or people, but they seldom have any sense of date or chronology. Pictures can provide an anchor to the *time* we are discussing in a lecture by portraying events or famous people from an era. A photograph of a newspaper front page with headlines "Fort Sumter Fired Upon" or "Lindbergh Lands" tells an audience *when* they are. A picture of Henry Ford's Model T, of a Lenin, or an Einstein, permits a lecturer, with a minimum of words, to place an audience in time. Comparative events—relating the publication of Vesalius' *Fabrica* to the death in the same year of Copernicus by a slide of either a Copernicus portrait or of a contemporary picture of the heliocentric solar system—will anchor both events in time. One can recall a social change like the industrial revolution with pictures of mills and mill workers before one presents material on the impact of the French revolution on medicine in France. In all of these examples, one should give a year or bracket of dates, but more critically, we can give our students some sense of what *else* was happening in the world as we discuss in detail what was happening in medical history.

As with time, most of our students have a limited sense of space and geography. Maps are valuable; they show the audience *where* things are happening. Historical political maps—the extent of the Roman empire, or the mini-state subdivisions of Renaissance Italy—place our medical history and illustrate in another way a context in which events occurred. Specialized cartography is extraordinarily valuable. The geographic distribution of a disease or its spread in time or the diffusion of a culture or a concept in space over time provides vivid imagery for which words can be no substitute.

The art representative of a period is both easy to make good slides from and is another way to again provide the surrounding, the setting, the context against which one can play the major theme of the medical issues of the time and place.

We frequently quote an author, describe the work of "the great person," refer to so-and-so's contributions, or philosophy, or influence, and so on. When one mentions a name, show a picture of the person. Try to use a picture that shows the person at the age they were when the "work" was done. If the lecture is focused as "the man and his work," show pictures of the man at work, and of the laboratory, clinic, or hospital where the work was done. If one is quoting historical figures, have their picture on the screen, so that it seems as if they are speaking while one is reading their "immortal words."

We refer to "classic texts" frequently in our lectures. Show a picture of the title page (especially if it is one of the early texts with illuminated title pages). When quoting from a book have the title page or the exact page being cited on the screen. Present the illusion that the audience is reading from the text. Where text citation is from the primary source—and particularly if one is quoting—show the manuscript page, the letter, the diary entry. If discussing "the work," show the laboratory notebook page, the original drawing, sketch, table, or graph.

This brings me to presenting historical data in modern formats—the bar or line graph, the table, the chart. Our students see every other subject, in basic and clinical science, at lectures, grand rounds, seminars, or scientific sessions, presented by data on slides. They are accustomed to following an argument from data given or presented that way. We can do the same thing.

First of all, tabular data are convincing by their familiarity, provided one keeps tables short, simple, and easy to read (table 1). Similarly, we can convert old written descriptions to a modern epidemiological format, as with Carter's data on the extrinsic incubation of yellow fever (fig. 1). We can assemble data from several sources and relate them to time and event variables, as with sick rates in the Royal Navy (fig. 2). Or, we can plot tabular data as graphs. The bar graph can be compelling, as with John Snow's data on cholera deaths as a function of the source of water (fig. 3). Replotted tabular data, like the famous Broad Street Pump report by Snow (fig. 4), not only clearly destroy the myth that this was the convincing experiment, but allows us to quote Snow when he says exactly that. And note, in figure 4, how we can relate this clearly plotted point source outbreak directly to the epidemiological theory our students are learning or have learned in other courses.

People and data lead to patients and to the care of patients. Students in the health professions are interested in patients, they are their reasons for entering the profession. Pictures of patients, whether bas-relief, sculpture, painting, or photograph, are available everywhere. Art and photography of patients and physicians or nurses are equally common. Not only do such pictures illuminate contemporary ideas of disease, trauma, or illness, they also bring discussion and examples of medical practice, or nursing care, or role representation to life. Here is an area where discussion of the picture itself provides the historical lesson.[4] The loving care of Jan Steen's seventeenth-century physician in "The Sick One" may be contrasted to Rowlandson's satirical "Dr. Double-dose" a century later. Whether one is discussing Jenner or McEwan, a photograph of a smallpox patient makes the listeners understand the horror of the disease. There are illustrations of trauma and surgical pro-

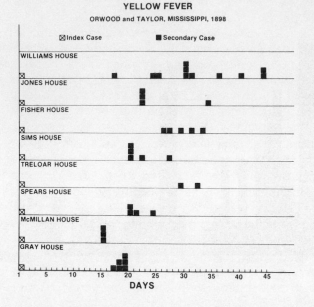

FIGURE 1. Index and secondary case data on yellow fever transmission, plotted from: H. Carter, "A note on the interval between infecting and secondary cases of yellow fever," *New Orleans Med. Surg. J.,* 1900, *52:* 617–36.

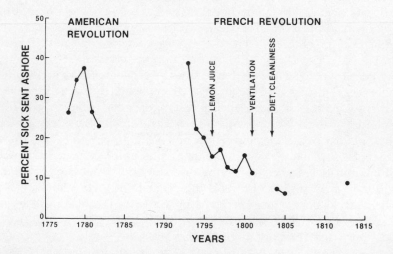

FIGURE 2. Assembled data, various sources, largely from G. Blane, "Health of the British Navy," *Med. Chirurg. Trans. (London),* 1815, *6:* 490–525.

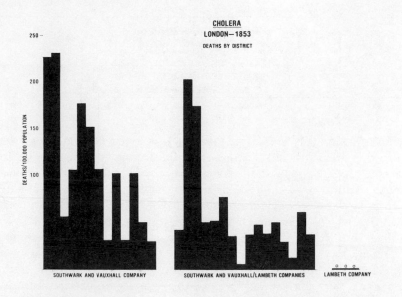

FIGURE 3. Bar graph of Table 6 in J. Snow, *On the Mode of Communication of Cholera* (London: John Churchill, 1855).

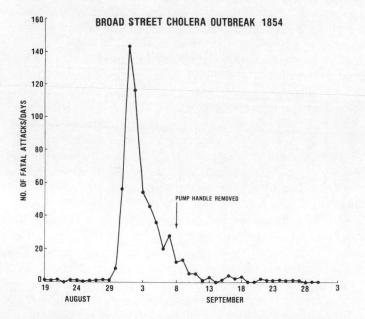

FIGURE 4. Line graph of Table 1 in J. Snow, *On the Mode of Communication of Cholera* (London: John Churchill, 1855).

TABLE 1. French Field Hospitals. Battles of the Frontiers

NINE FIELD HOSPITALS
NOVEMBER 1792–MARCH 1793

TOTAL FEVER PATIENTS	1752
TOTAL FEVER DEATHS	375
21% DEATH RATE	

Adapted from D. M. Vess, *Medical Revolution in France* (Florida State University, 1975), p. 139.

cedures from nearly every age. Study figure 5, von Gersdorff's picture of an amputation (the first such ever printed). Note how surgeon, assistant, and patient are posed, the previous patient in the rear, the handling of the instruments. Could one describe this only in words? How better to present the history of antisepsis than by a series of slides showing surgeons at the operating table as their dress changed from street clothes and bare hands to masks and gloves, to the sterile green mummies of today?

There are times when the lecturer does not want to show a picture or a graph, but wishes the audience to direct its attention to the speaker. This is the place for a blank slide—exposed film in the regular 2 x 2 mount. This trick should be better known, as it permits a lecturer to have a dark screen while putting a period to a part of a lecture, summarizing particular points, or permitting an interlude for discussion or questions. Using the blank slide avoids the distraction of a white screen and stops the pernicious and distracting "projector-on—projector-off" interruptions common to many speakers.

If one cannot or chooses not to illustrate a point, then the key word slide (table 2) is often useful. This has the virtue of imprinting the major themes visually and can also serve as the "lecture notes" for the speaker who can deliver impromptu comments while not forgetting any important topic. A reinforcement is sequential highlighting, in which a separate slide is made for each key word, colored to highlight (in yellow) the key word, while leaving all the other words (in blue) subdued but still on the screen. The student will be struck by the highlighted word, but is still receiving information "subliminally" from the subdued words still on the screen.

Much of the history of medicine we wish to teach our students is an aspect of social, economic, or political history. These approaches can be illustrated. Pictures of legislators, farm or factory workers, city streets, people in wealth or poverty, men, women, and children about their daily occupations, hospitals, poorhouses—a thousand things: there are paintings or caricatures or photographs of them all. The political cartoon, for example, is a very useful illustration for these topics. Accompanying graphs can be made relating disease to social change.[5]

There are ways to illustrate even certain philosophies or theories.

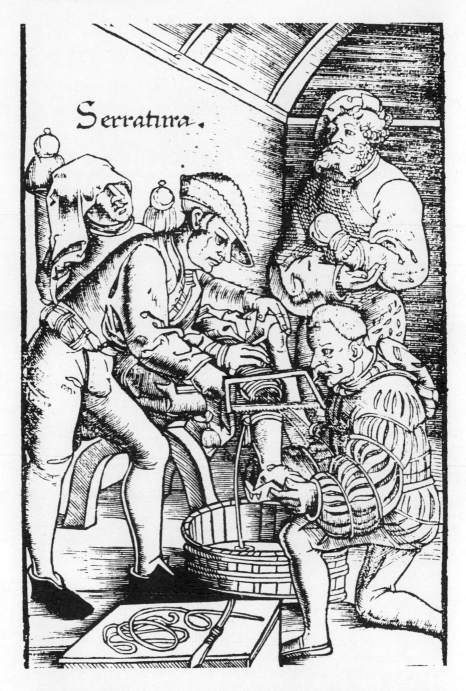

FIGURE 5. "Amputation" from Hans von Gersdorff, *Feldtbuch der Wundartzney* (Strasburg, 1517).

TABLE 2. Key Word Slide (Used in Lecture to List Clinical Specialties in Order of Usefulness to Military Medicine)

THE MEDICAL OFFICER
DIRECT SUPPORT IN BATTLE
SURGERY
PREVENTIVE MEDICINE
INFECTIOUS DISEASES
TROPICAL MEDICINE
ENVIRONMENTAL MEDICINE
PSYCHIATRY

Figures 6 and 7 show simple graphics that outline for the student the interactions of Greek natural philosophy and the applications to the humoral theory.

A word on films and video tapes. They have their place—especially as short clips of two to three minutes within a lecture—and are always useful as supplemental material. I prefer not to use filmed "dramas" because the script and actors take up too much time; the historical content per unit time is too thin. Since I prefer to have a live lecturer in front of an audience, I would not recommend substituting film, no matter how good. But this is a point of personal preference.

Finally, how *many* slides should one use in a fifty-minute lecture? This is obviously a matter of taste, style, topic, and availability. I use between 120 and 150 slides per fifty-minute lecture, drawn from our collection of over 7000 slides (to which we are still adding). People can grasp the contents in a picture in a fraction of a second.[6] To explain a graph or discuss a particular picture obviously takes longer, but should never exceed a minute. One has only to attend the ten-minute presentations at a scientific meeting to see how much data can be presented and assimilated if slides are properly used.

Now, how does one *get* all these pictures?[7] First and foremost, one has to *think* visually. In the same way that we read in our field and collect new insights and new information, one must always be on the alert for a new picture. I can put it no more helpfully. If one does not *think* illustration, one will not "see" the material that surrounds us. A word of caution: except for a rare lecture that one plans from illustration, for example, "Hospital Architecture Through the Ages," one should prepare the lecture first and illustrate it afterwards.[8] To plan a historical lecture around "pretty pictures" is too often to give a shallow (but well-illustrated) lecture. In another context, a review of the popular science books and television programs of Carl Sagan puts it succinctly: "It is a short step from using beautiful pictures to illustrate articles to using science as a peg on which to hang beautiful pictures."[9] In this context, the present essay (and the spoken version with slides) is a "how-to-do-it" talk; it is not a historical lecture or paper.

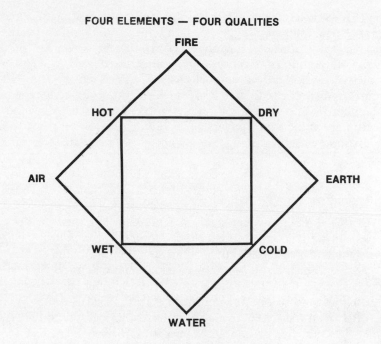

FIGURE 6. Simple graphics of Greek view of organization of nature.

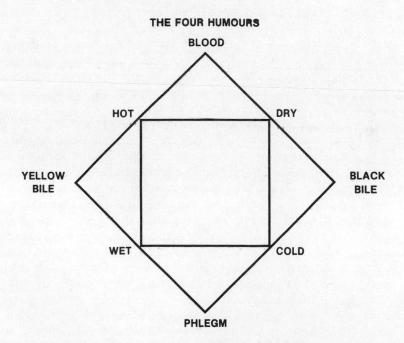

FIGURE 7. Application of Greek ontology to a theory of physiology.

This said, let me briefly describe only a few of the sources of material. The following suggestions only hint at the kind and variety of material that is available. Fox and Terry should be consulted for a fine review of the sources.[10] There is a magnificent archive in the History of Medicine Division at the National Library of Medicine.[11] The National Archive and Records Center has excellent topic-area collections well catalogued.[12] The Center of Photographic Images of Medicine and Health Care at the State University of New York, Stony Brook, is, as of this writing, just beginning but promises to be a major source of material.[13]

"Coffee-table" books are extraordinarily helpful.[14] A word of caution: one can trust the annotation of books like those by Lyons and Petrucelli or Herrlinger, or of meticulously researched series like those by Horizon, American Heritage, or Time-Life; but there are popular books on the market, with excellent pictures, in. which it is wise to verify the attribution, date, title, or artist of the illustrations.

Biographies and autobiographies usually have pictures of their subjects, and often have illustrations of their work, their laboratories, contemporaries, and so on. Accounts of a disease or a scientific discipline are often well illustrated as are specialized monographs on a medical topic.[15] Do not overlook popular magazines, in particular those written especially for audiences interested in history.[16] Historical atlases are invaluable, and here you will find not only the geographical and political cartography, but very often also the specialized cartography illustrating the diffusion of a culture or the distributions of a technology.[17] Search for collections of photographs of an era or a place; these are becoming more common as iconographic monographs.[18]

It is obvious that journal articles, textbooks, monographs, and other professional publications should be explored. A picture of apparatus, a kymograph tracing, or the photograph or sketch of a patient or operation are splendidly evocative of the science or medical practice of the time. Local hospital and university archives, newspaper files, historical societies, and government offices often contain pictorial material that is of both local and national interest; not infrequently these collections will have important pictures that the custodians do not know they own.

The issue of copyright is not a problem for the teacher. The law and its present interpretations make clear that a teacher may make one copy of material for use in teaching in a nonprofit institution. The fair use restrictions will not hamper such teachers in reasonable use of copyrighted material.[19]

I find no better summary for my argument than the words of Max Fisch discussing Vesalius:

The picture is itself a statement. Moreover, the picture says something . . . which cannot be said in words; so that it does not merely fix the meanings of the words . . . but makes a contribution all its own to a total meaning which the words could not convey alone. This relation between words and pictures is mutual; for pictures also suffer from ambiguity, and though words cannot say what the picture can, they can restrict the range of the picture's possible meanings. When words and pictures seem to say the same thing, that is an illusion produced by the interpretation of each by the other, so that together they convey an integral meaning. . . .[20]

Acknowledgements. Mrs. P. DuBose has been invaluable in manuscript preparation. Mrs. F. Langley in graphic arts and Mr. J. Swope in photography have taught me and provided my material for years. Mrs. C. Unger guided me to many of the references cited.

Notes

1. G. Cornstock et al., *Television and Human Behavior* (New York: Columbia University Press, 1978); see *Time,* 16 June 1980, p. 59, for a typical statement of the present conventional wisdom.

2. See topic areas in D. A. Norman, *Memory and Attention* (New York: Wiley, 1969).

3. R. M. Yerkes and J. D. Dodson, "The relation of strength of stimulus to rapidity of habit formation," *J. Comp. Neurol. Psychol.,* 1908, *18:* 459–82.

4. The image as a historical document is discussed by D. M. Fox and J. Terry, "Photography and the self image of American physicians: 1880–1920," *Bull. Hist. Med.,* 1978, *52:* 435–57; see also the exhaustive study by S. B. Burns, "Early medical photography in America," *New York State Med. J.,* 1979, *79:* 788–795, 943–947, 1256–1268, 1931–1938, and 1980, *80:* 270–282, 1444–1469.

5. E. H. Kass, "Infectious disease and social change," *J. Inf. Dis.,* 1971, *123:* 110–14.

6. G. Sperling, "The information available in brief visual presentations," *Psychol. Monographs,* 1960, *74:* no. 498.

7. There are a number of directories. See B. Eastwood, *Directory of Audio-Visual Sources* (New York: Science History Publications, 1979), with its 41 pages, 543 entries. The journal *Picturescope* (Washington, D.C., Special Libraries Association) announces new collections and archives quarterly. Dover Publications, 180 Varick Street, New York, N.Y. 10014 is a good source of inexpensive but good quality reprints of collections of photographs and drawings.

8. J. D. Thompson and G. Goldin, *The Hospital* (New Haven: Yale University Press, 1975), is the best modern illustrated source for architectural study, especially the first 203 pages by Goldin.

9. E. Edelson, "Carl Sagan's dilemma," *The Dial,* 1980, *1:* 7–11.

10. Fox and Terry, "Photography."

11. Communications should be addressed to Mrs. Lucinda Keister, National Library of Medicine, Bethesda, Maryland 20209.

12. National Archives and Records Service National Audiovisual Center, Washingon, D.C. 20409.

13. "Announcement," *Bull. Hist. Med.,* 1978, *52:* 462.

14. There are hundreds of such books on the market. The following list directs attention to those that I have found to have good quality reproductions and to be especially useful in my own work: A. S. Lyons and R. J. Petrucelli, *Medicine: An Illustrated History* (New York: Harry N. Abrams, 1978); R. Herrlinger, *History of Medical Illustration from Antiquity to A.D. 1600* (New York: Medicina Rara, 1970); S. G. F. Brandon, ed., *Milestones of History* (New York: W. W. Norton, 1971); C. Zigrosser, *Medicine and the Artist,* (New York: Dover, 1970); C. D. Haagerson and W. E. B. Lloyd, *One Hundred Years of Medicine* (New York: Sheridan, 1943); E. Ackerknecht, *The World of Asclepios: A History of Medicine in Objects* (Stuttgart: Huber, 1966); F. Marti-Ibanez, *Epic of Medicine* (New York: Potter, 1962); The *Horizon Book* series is exceptional: N. Kotkar, *The Middle Ages* (New York: Houghton Mifflin, 1967); L. B. Smith, *The Elizabethan World* (New York: Houghton Mifflin, 1967); J. H. Plumb, *The Renaissance* (New York: Doubleday, 1961); J. C. Herold, *Napoleon* (New York: Harper & Row, 1963).

15. N. Longmate, *King Cholera* (London: Hamilton, 1966); P. Baldry, *The Battle against Bacteria: A History of the Development of Antibacterial Drugs* (London: Cambridge University Press, 1976); H. J. Parish, *A History of Immunization* (Edinburgh: E. & S. Livingstone, 1965); G. Majno, *The Heal-*

ing Hand (Cambridge: Harvard University Press, 1975); P. Huard, *Sciences, Médecine, Pharmacie de la Révolution á l'Empire: 1789–1815* (Paris: R. DaCosta, 1970).

16. Representative publications are: *American Heritage, American History Illustrated, British Heritage, Smithsonian, National Geographic, Historic Preservation.*

17. Again, there are many such publications. Among those I have found most helpful are: *Historical Atlas of the World* (New York: Barnes & Noble, 1970); J. G. Bartholomew, *Twentieth Century Citizen's Atlas* (London, 1900); G. Barraclough, *The Times Atlas of World History* (London: Times Books, 1978); R. R. Palmer, *Historical Atlas* (New York: Rand-McNally, 1965); C. McEvedy, *The Penguin Atlas of Modern History to 1815* (London: Penguin, n.d.); O. Bjorklund, *Historical Atlas of the World* (New York: Barnes & Noble, 1970).

18. Among many such studies are the excellent collections of: A. Trachtenberg, *The American Image: 1860–1960* (New York: Pantheon, 1979); T. Burke, *The Streets of London* (London: Batsford, 1940); A. Smith and J. Thompson, *Street Life in London* (1877; reprint ed., London: Blom, 1969); L. C. B. Seaman, *Life in Victorian London* (London: Batsford, 1973).

19. See Public Law 94–553, Section 107. Extended discussion and explanations of the intent of Congress may be found in: *Reproduction of Copyrighted Works by Educators and Librarians, Circular R–21* (Washington, D.C.: Library of Congress, 1978); *Copyright and Educational Media* (Washington, D.C.: Association of Media Producers; Association for Educational Communications and Technology, 1977); *The New Copyright Law* (Washington, D.C.: National Education Association, 1977).

20. M. H. Fisch, "Vesalius and his book," *Bull. Med. Lib. Assoc,* 1943, *31:* 208–21.

SOME EXPERIENCES WITH SEMINARS IN THE HISTORY OF MEDICINE

Saul Jarcho

This presentation has three parts. The first is a narrative of experiences and observations that extend over fifty-and-a-half years, approximately from the spring of 1930 to the autumn of 1980. The second contains inferences derived from these experiences. The final part hazards some speculations about the teaching and the practice of the history of medicine in this country today and during the next two decades.

In 1930, as a senior student at the College of Physicians and Surgeons, Columbia University, I attended a seminar in the history of medicine conducted by C.N.B. Camac (1868–1940). At that time Dr. Camac was assistant professor of clinical medicine. Early in his career he had been one of Osler's assistant residents, hence his interest in medical history may well have been of Oslerian origin.[1] His writings include papers on clinical subjects and two books on the history of medicine.[2]

Dr. Camac's pleasant seminar was conducted in a small periodicals room in the college library.[3] I remember almost nothing at all about it— neither the season during which it was held, nor the frequency or number of the sessions. The room could hardly have held more than a dozen students, but I do not remember which of my classmates attended nor do I remember ever discussing the subject matter with any of them. I have the faint and fading recollection that Dr. Camac was the sole speaker and that the menu was a simple introduction to some famous medical writings. I do not remember the name of a single author who was discussed. If I then knew that the library of the school possessed a collection of medical classics, which had been deposited there by John G. Curtis (1844–1913), a professor of physiology long deceased, I rediscovered the fact eight years later.

Of Dr. Camac's civil and well-intentioned efforts it can be said that if, as far as anyone knows, they left no permanent impression, they at the same time alienated no one—so far as anyone knows. As Oliver Goldsmith wrote in his review of Auenbrugger's treatise on percussion of the chest, "If it cannot cure, it can do you no harm."[4]

In the respect that I have mentioned, Dr. Camac's mild seminars were superior to the off-putting pedagogy that probably every one of us has experienced in one subject or another at one time or another. It should also be noticed that the college had made available the curricular time, the room, and the learned instructor. This, as I have said, was in 1930.

In 1934–35, in Baltimore, Henry Sigerist conducted a seminar on Thomas Sydenham. Although it was dangerous rather than burdensome to walk from my office in the department of pathology diagonally across Wolfe and Monument Streets to the Welch Library, absorption in morbid anatomy left time for no more than one or two visits to the Sigerist seminar. Moreover, the Department of Pathology possessed *Virchows Archiv,* beginning with the first volume. It also had the very recent tradition of William Welch and the presence of William MacCallum and Arnold Rich.

Sigerist proved to be a vivacious and stimulating teacher. He not only brought original texts to the seminar, and had them read aloud, but he used them as an introduction to problems in clinical medicine. Indeed, his seminar was part of the third-year course in medicine. There could be no doubt of the interest that Dr. Sigerist aroused in the participants. It was valuable to have seen him in action. *Virgilium vidi tantum.*

In 1936 I became instructor in pathology at the College of Physicians and Surgeons, the school at which I had attended Dr. Camac's seminars. Instruction in the history of medicine was no longer being given. In 1941 I suggested to the assistant dean that it would be desirable to establish a seminar. His reply was substantially as follows: "Since the students' time is all taken up, you could not give the seminars in the daytime. Since all the classrooms are in use, none of the college buildings will be available. But I want you to know that I'm with you all the way." [5]

With this hyperthermic encouragement, seminars were instituted. They were given at night in a dormitory building and continued until interrupted by military duty in the autumn of 1942. Eight meetings were held in five months. The average attendance must have been about twenty. The participants were mainly undergraduate medical students and young instructors. In most instances the subjects for presentation were suggested to prospective speakers and the basic textual material was supplied to them. For obvious reasons the subject matter leaned toward problems of military and naval medicine, such as the work of Richard Brocklesby, Lord Anson's scorbutic voyages, and the recent destruction of the water supply of Singapore by the Japanese. All the materials were in English.

There is no clear evidence that these seminars left a persistent impression, although one student showed mild continuing interest. The unhelpful assistant dean later became dean of an eminent Eastern medical school and wrote a book on medical education, which was published in 1974.

In December 1946, Frederic D. Zeman (1894–1970) and I instituted a seminar in the history of medicine at the Mount Sinai Hospital in New York. Zeman was the prototype of the learned, sagacious, and kindly internist. During the First World War, he had served as a junior member of the Empyema Commission. He later became a leader in the new field of geriatrics and he contributed importantly to the history of that subject. In addition, his knowledge of geology had led him to study the geological contributions of William Withering.[6] In 1946, Dr. Zeman and I were members of the attending staff at Mount Sinai Hospital. We had strong support from the chief of the medical service, George Baehr (1887–1978), a pupil of the famous Emanuel Libman and a man who had had extensive personal experience with historic events.[7] The seminars were given monthly, from eight to eleven months a year from 1946 to 1951, to an audience of thirty to fifty persons. The speakers usually, but by no means always, were members of the house staff or junior members of the visiting staff. Quite often, as with the Columbia seminar previously described, it was necessary to suggest subjects to the younger speakers and to provide the source material half-cooked.[8]

It was otherwise with the discussions and the discussants. The latter were apt to be members of the senior staff, or physicians who served the outpatient clinics, or volunteer physicians, or members of the medical public at large. And here was the big surprise. Numbers of discussants were erudite refugees from the distressed cities and countries of Europe. There were men and women from Prague and Jena and Warsaw and Amsterdam and Berlin and Munich and Florence, and many from Vienna. These people had studied with the great masters and in some instances were eminent in their own right. They were well educated. They had seen much and had lived through much, and they valued history.

In 1951 we had a new chief-of-service. The seminars did not survive. Apart from announcements in the *Bulletin of the History of Medicine,* a single published article is the sole memorial of their existence.[9] There is no distinct evidence that any young participant in the seminars derived from them a permanent or productive interest in the history of medicine. On the day or the week after a session, it was not rare to meet some member of the audience who might say, "That was an interesting paper we had on What-Was-His-Name?" a remark which suggests how little had been remembered.

In subsequent years a seminar or lecture series was set up at Columbia by Dickinson Richards, with help from Paul Klemperer and George Rosen. It can hardly have lasted more than two or three years.

What can we make of apparently random experiences such as I have described? More precisely, what observations can be registered and what inferences drawn?

I have avoided defining the seminar, since it is difficult to demarcate. Seminars in the history of medicine often resemble, or are almost identical to, local medico-historical clubs. In the United States they tend to be informal, which does not preclude seriousness of intent. Extra-academic seminars tend to be short lived and to leave fragmentary records or none at all. The most persistent organizations in the general category under discussion are probably not seminars but university historical clubs, such as the Johns Hopkins Medical History Club, which is now approaching its centennial, and which doubtless has inspired the creation of clubs and seminars in many parts of the United States and elsewhere.[10]

Both inside universities and outside universities, the approval of persons in authority is by no means essential to the existence of the seminar, but unquestionably it can be helpful; approval is likely to make available the meager physical facilities that are needed.

I think it has been demonstrated that the informal seminar need not be inferior, qualitatively or quantitatively, to its formal collegiate analogues, and that persons who stand at or beyond the periphery of an institution may prove to be valuable participants.

The seminar, then, is a valid alternative pedagogic method and, when it exists apart from a university, may have larger and more diverse audiences than can be reached by standard academic evangelism. Like many other educational enterprises, it is difficult to judge. Indeed, part of its effect may be unobtrusive, invisible, or delayed; hence its continued existence may be an act of faith. While a historical seminar or a medical history club is to be expected in a medical school, when it exists in an independent medical center it may be an oasis in a anti-humanistic desert.

If we discuss the teaching of the history of medicine, we cannot avoid wondering who henceforth will become a medical historian. What will be the source of new physician-historians of medicine during the two final decades of this century?

On the present occasion I do not make bold to consider otherwise than incidentally the nonphysicians or nonscientists who undertake to write the history of medicine, especially the nonphysician social historians. These men and women are mainly historians or sociologists who have chosen medicine, or some part of medicine, as their subject matter. The supply of such persons presumably is influenced by whatever factors affect the supply of historians and sociologists in general. It is conceivable and not improbable that hard times may drive, and may have driven, some members of these groups into medical history, where they have the opportunity to make an illuminating contribution.

The belief is now current that, in addition to the nonphysician historians of medicine whose writings satisfy the best contemporary criterion and have gained widespread esteem, there are at least a few whose writings show grave weaknesses, especially ignorance, credulity, misunderstanding, and a bias against physicians.[11] Whether this is true or not—and I consider the allegation not unfounded—there is room for a survey by responsible scholars.

Some social historians have been accused of belittling the role of the physician in medical history. Such an attitude need not infuriate the orthodox physician-historian, since it may merely express an alternative concept of cause; namely, that historical developments are usually due to conditions, especially social and economic conditions, rather than to individual men and women. This simplistic concept is the tattered bequest of Karl Marx, whether its present-day advocates are aware of the fact or not. Debate on this aspect might be improved by reference to Aristotle's *Metaphysics*.

For the physician-historian of medicine, professional training is now available in university departments. One problem is the supply of candidates. It happens occasionally nowadays that a clinical instructor or professor changes directions, takes formal training in historiography, and then teaches the history of medicine. Some persons enter this category after having been the victims of academic assassination. Others have found clinical or laboratory work or administration unsatisfying and are happier as medical historians. Many others seek the historical origins of their own specialities and problems.

As we now know, before the specialization and professionalization of American medical historians, an important body of medico-historical writing—indeed, almost the entire product—was provided by the practicing physician, who was often a person trained in the Greco-Roman or Hebrew classics, or both, who turned to the history of medicine, studied it, and wrote about it. In the ranks of this regiment marched Krumbhaar, Long, Castiglioni, Friedenwald, Major, Clendening, and a thousand of their contemporaries and predecessors. To the perceptive treatment of this subject by Genevieve Miller in her Fielding H. Garrison Lecture, I shall merely add, outside her theme, that Thucydides and Edward Gibbon can be classed as amateurs as well.[12]

Over the men and women who seek to be today's physician-historians a double threat now hangs. The continuing necrosis of American preliminary education has yielded ignorance of ancient and modern languages, inadequate contact with scholarship, and flaccidity in the use of English. A minor collateral result is the opinion, which I have heard in staff rooms, that "nothing worthwhile is being written in foreign languages, anyhow."

A second and newer threat is the requirement of triennial clinical reexamination and requalification, with the prospect of endless brush-up courses and endless grubbing for credits and points. This innovation, so impressive to meliorists, journalists, bureaucrats, and perhaps to ambitious members of Congress, menaces an important source of medical historians. Who can study Galen while perpetually taking courses and examinations in ultra-cardiography or thaumatology? Our last recourse may yet be the physician who was educated and trained abroad.

Acknowledgements. Mrs. Paul Weaver, Mr. Donald Clyde, and Mr. Dennis Gaffney assisted in the collection and verification of facts presented in this paper.

Notes

1. As might be expected, Camac is mentioned repeatedly in Harvey Cushing's biography of Osler.
2. C.N.B. Camac, *Epoch-making Contributions to Medicine, Surgery, and the Allied Sciences* (Philadelphia: Saunders, 1909); and idem, *Imhotep to Harvey: The Backgrounds of the History of Medicine* (New York: Hoeber, 1931). The seminars are described on pp. xiii–xvi.
3. Additional information will be found in G. Miller, "Medical history," in R. L. Numbers, ed., *The Education of American Physicians: Historical Essays* (Berkeley: University of California Press, 1980), pp. 290–308; see, especially, pp. 301–6.
4. The review appeared in the *Public Ledger,* a London newspaper, on 27 August 1761. See S. Jarcho, "A review of Auenbrugger's *Inventum Novum,* attributed to Oliver Goldsmith," *Bull. Hist. Med.,* 1959, *33:* 470–74.
5. Substantially, not verbatim.
6. F. D. Zeman, "William Withering as a mineralogist: the story of witherite," *Bull. Hist. Med.,* 1950, *24:* 530–38.
7. *Inter alia,* he had participated in the efforts of the Red Cross to stem typhus in Serbia during World War I, he had been imprisoned by the Austrian army and had written a paper during his imprisonment, he had studied pathology with Ludwig Aschoff and pharmacology with J.E.O. Schmiedeberg, and he had served during World War II as chief medical officer of civilian defense.
8. Sometimes the material that we furnished half-cooked was dished up half-baked.
9. *Bull. Hist. Med.,* 1947, *21* to 1951, *25;* H. Janowitz, "Newly discovered letters concerning William Beaumont, Alexis St. Martin, and the American Fur Company," *Bull. Hist. Med.,* 1948, *22:* 822–32.
10. It is to be hoped that this organization will be given the thorough history that it so obviously deserves. It would be interesting to know whether the club at Johns Hopkins was influenced by the seminars in history that were given during the earliest years of the university.
11. Recent evidences of dissatisfaction with the work of nonphysician historians of medicine will be found in the editorial, "Medical history without medicine," *J. Hist. Med.,* 1980, *35:* 5–7, and a book review by L. G. Stevenson, in *Bull. Hist. Med.,* 1980, *54:* 131–40.
12. G. Miller, "In praise of amateurs: medical history in America before Garrison," *Bull. Hist. Med.,* 1973, *47:* 586–615.

TEACHING MEDICAL HISTORY TO MEDICAL STUDENTS: THE MCGILL EXPERIENCE, 1966–1981*

Don G. Bates

Fifteen years ago, the role of the history of medicine in the education of medical students was moot. Should students be obliged to take it? What should be the form and content of what was taught? What are the purposes that such teaching should fulfill? [1]

My own attitude at that time was that there is no single, right answer to those questions.[2] Fifteen years of teaching the subject at McGill University and conversing with my colleagues from other centers has strengthened my conviction that a pluralistic approach is the only way and that generalizations are hazardous. Two variables have a profound effect on what transpires: local conditions and the particularities of the professor. Because of this, what follows is not a general or theoretical discussion of teaching the history of medicine at a medical center, but a fairly personal account of the events at McGill's medical school since the inception of a department of the history of medicine in 1966.

At that time, the local conditions were particularly favorable to the subject on a number of counts. Most important, there was a strong tradition of interest in the history of medicine that had already existed for almost half a century. The centerpiece of this was the Osler Library, rich in both symbol and substance, endowed with Sir William Osler's magic and his fame.[3] Moreover, the library had been nurtured for thirty years by the corporeal expression of Osler's love of books and history, W. W. Francis. This Oslerian tradition formed a focal point in the McGill medical faculty's vision of its own past and present as a leading North American institution in medical research and teaching.[4] It seemed clear at the time that if the history of medicine at McGill did nothing more than nourish that spiritual font of collegial pride it would be justified, and supported, and that anyone coming to the post of historian of medicine had a responsibility to see that his subject did nothing less.[5]

The second local condition, much indebted to the first, was the existence of outstanding physical facilities. Partly by design and partly

*This paper was not presented at the symposium but was submitted on invitation in the spring of 1981.

by architectural accident, these facilities mixed elegantly appointed rooms, which made tradition visible, with a substantial amount of undifferentiated space, which could be used for expansion. These happy circumstances came about, in turn, because a historian was dean of medicine just when these facilities were being planned, and he played a decisive role in the shape they took and the very fact that they materialized.[6]

In the face of all this it was hardly surprising that McGill University was able to raise a development grant to start a department and to establish an endowed chair in the history of medicine when the grant ended. Given this situation, it would have required more than ordinary maladroitness for someone not to have flourished.

The point of these remarks is not merely to pass out bouquets or to make a perfunctory tip of the cap, even though acknowledgements in the direction of the university and one's predecessors are well deserved. Nor do I wish to suggest that these exceptional institutional supports were responsible for the direction that the history of medicine at McGill has taken in the past decade and a half. Rather, I wish to underline the importance of a secure institutional base in permitting those concerned with the subject to explore and develop it, and to reach out to professional historians, medical faculty administrators, amateur physician-historians, medical students, and many other sectors of the university with the confidence that no one of them would, by itself, be the source of the program's continued existence. Such a secure and flexible setting is in the very best traditions of a university, and it is unfortunate that not all medical centers in North America that have given a place to medical history have done so wholeheartedly and with a view to establishing a firm foundation.

In 1966, then, there was a solid tradition of medical history: a well-organized library in the process of providing first-rate teaching and research facilities; the establishment of a fully constituted (albeit one-man) department in the medical faculty; a development grant; and an endowed chair in the offing. Given these, where did medical history at McGill go, and why? To answer this, I must turn to the relevant events of the next fifteen years and, reluctantly, to the person most directly involved.

I say "reluctantly," not only because this resort to autobiography seems a doubtful undertaking, but because it is embarrassing to admit that the security of the institutional commitment to medical history just described was, at first, considerably offset by my own insecurity. There were many doubts: doubts about my own competence as a historian, conflicts over my professional identity as historian *versus* physician, misgivings about the real value of the history of medicine in a medical school, feelings of being marginal with respect to my medical colleagues, and a considerable sense of isolation from collegial exchange of any kind.

In retrospect, I suspect that it was these doubts, as much as political calculation, which caused me to rule out the further development of the department along purely history-of-medicine lines.[7] Looking back, I can now conceive that the department might have been granted some growth strictly within the confines of medical history. But in those early years I was convinced that an expansion of this sort was virtually impossible and that, if I wanted to end my isolation and to build a context for my subject, I would have to broaden the disciplinary base of the department.

Whatever the role of internal misgivings, there were many external factors to conspire with my enthusiasm for a broadened disciplinary base. One obvious ally was the history of science, which was, in 1966, struggling to gain more visible support and expression at McGill. Although I was not entirely convinced, in principle, of the merits of such a liaison, it seemed pragmatically sound to combine forces with history of science advocates. A combination of budgetary constraints and the lack of conviction of a senior university administrator, however, thwarted the aims of our coalition and when, several years later, the history of science at McGill gained considerable strength, the history of medicine had already gone off in another direction.[8]

In retrospect, it was probably just as well that that venture did not succeed. For the fact was that, within the subject of medicine itself, I had always had a stronger liking for the clinical than for the basic sciences. Hence, although the history of science, as it was still being pursued in the mid-1960s, might have seemed to offer a natural home for the devotee of intellectual history that I then was, I maintained the clinician's ambivalence about the equation of medical practice with medical science, along with a conviction that the historiography of medicine for the past fifty years—Henry Sigerist, Richard Shryock, and Erwin Ackerknecht to the contrary notwithstanding—had been unduly oriented to the history of medical sciences, in imitation of professional medicine's excessive claims to be based largely on science.[9]

Coincident with those abortive efforts to reach out to the history of science was a growing, if not wholehearted, interest in the social history of medicine. Large-scale social forces, in a fairly materialistic if not truly Marxist framework, seemed to furnish far more powerful tools for the analysis and critique of medicine's past than the intellectual history which, until then, I had by preference pursued in my research and reflected in my teaching.

Also pushing me in the direction of social history were two circumstances related to the late sixties and early seventies. One was the growing social consciousness of students. Although probably not much more numerous then than they are in the classes of the 1980s, the socially active students of the time were sounding a dominant note that was rippling across the values and beliefs of the student body at large.

Let me pause, for a moment, to comment on this particular phenomenon. Over the years I have come to appreciate that student preferences are complex and their reactions difficult to interpret. These reactions were never thoroughly measured at McGill in any scientific way, but could be gauged nevertheless from a number of sources.

It is my impression, for example, that about 25 to 35 percent of our students respond favorably to what I have called the large-scale, social-forces model of historical treatment. A decidedly larger constituency of first-year students would vote for the history of medicine as the history of the medical sciences presented in a fairly "internalistic" way. A similar or possibly even larger number (these categories not necessarily being mutually exclusive) would probably be happiest with a great-men, great-discoveries, great-events approach since this much more narrative, individualistic, and largely uncomplicated perspective accords best with students' own personal experiences and idealized view of the world they have come from and the professional life they aspire to.

This proportional composition, which I have reason to believe remains quite stable over many years, should not be confused with the often-observed variations from year to year in the dominant personality of particular classes.[10] This much more variable, even fickle, character of a class does not necessarily reflect the views of the majority but comes from the fact that those students who reflect the trends and fads in the larger society become the creators of class opinion, while others who sense that their views are at variance with the current orthodoxy keep quiet and go along to a considerable extent. As a result, the dominant posture may vary from class to class, while the underlying mix of views and outlooks remains surprisingly static. If, as I believe, these mechanisms are at work, generalizations about whole classes of medical students, as to their world-views and preferences, are of doubtful validity, despite these students' well-known homogeneity in other respects.

But if this is a valid insight it is also hindsight. In the late sixties, I too was influenced by the mood that was dominating the class and I too was responding to the prevailing themes in the larger society, just as the class opinion-leaders were doing. The Vietnam War, student unrest, drugs, hippies, the New Left, women's lib, environmentalism, social activism, and the rest of the social phenomena of those years were bringing fundamental changes to the outlooks and attitudes of all of us.

This brings me to the second circumstance that pushed me in the direction of social history. During those years, Quebec itself was in the throes of major change in the politics and social structure of health care, culminating in a blueprint for the extensive reorganization of health care delivery and its institutions, a doctor's strike, and the establishment of one of the most complete, government-run medical insurance plans in the Western world.[11] When one recalls that these events were coupled with the activism of an aroused and socially aware student body, it need hardly be added that the "relevance" of the social aspects of medicine was self-evident in the McGill medical community at that time. Indeed, although student activism has since died down, and the passions aroused at the time have subsided, the continuing evolution of health care in Quebec, from that day to this, has meant a steady pressure upon medical educators and students to acknowledge and to take account of the social dimensions of medicine.[12]

This general atmosphere encouraged the social orientation that the course was then developing. In addition, my own participation in other activities such as curriculum planning, the teaching of the social aspects of present-day medicine, and the assisting of students in the development of a storefront clinic in a medically underserviced part of Montreal all had a strongly reinforcing effect on my own interest in the social context in which the practice of medicine takes place.

The practical outcome of all this, however, was fairly modest. The survey course in the history of medicine (taught then, as it still is, as a required course of twenty-four hours to first-year medical students) was constructed chiefly out of the material of Owsei Temkin's lectures at Hopkins, but largely from the course given in the School of Public Health, which was oriented to the social dimensions, and not from the course given to Hopkins medical students, which was focused more on the history of the basic sciences.[13]

As has been said, however, the commitment to social history was not wholehearted, or perhaps I should say, not comprehensive. On the one hand, I felt comfortable with, even stimulated by, a vision of the world that was explained in terms of large-scale, amoral, social forces machinating away without much regard for individual conscience, conscious beliefs, talents, or efforts: social forces that were, in addition, more or less grounded on a materialistic base. At the same time, such a world-view seemed unable to account for, or at least was a very tenuously related to, much of the activity of the healer which is so personal, so individual, and so doubtfully deducible from such a macrocosmic perspective. In other words, the typical approach of the social sciences seemed to fail, as the basic sciences seemed to fail, to do full justice to the nature of the healing act.

Upon this confused setting was superimposed yet another circumstance, not particularly related to the others. This was my introduction to medical anthropology through a then McGill colleague, John Janzen.

Even while still at Hopkins, the study of the history of disease in past centuries, combined with an acquaintance with some of the professors in the School of Public Health who were working in developing countries, had suggested that the past experience of European and North American countries with the major infectious diseases might be profitably compared with the present-day experience of other countries where these same or similar diseases still prevail. An abortive effort to spend some time in Ethiopia and a successful one to work temporarily on the Labrador coast in 1968, were expressions, in part, of this interest.

The ground was well prepared, therefore, for my exposure to the work of Janzen who, for five years, had been in Zaire studying native healing practices and beliefs. The most tangible consequences of our collaboration were two one-term graduate seminars in anthropology in 1970 and 1971: the first on the interaction between Western and indigenous medicine in several countries; the second, a careful analysis of specific case histories alternating between those supplied by Janzen from his field notes in Zaire, and those supplied by myself from patients seen in the student storefront clinic in Montreal.[14]

These experiences, combined with attendance for several years at the annual medical anthropology meetings, strengthened my belief that a fruitful link between anthropology and medical history could be forged; and led, eventually, to the appointment of Margaret Lock, a cultural anthropologist with a special interest in medicine, to our department.

Let me try to explain what I believe those links to be. The most obvious, of course, is that the history of medicine is, among other things, a comparative study of medicine that adds to our insight of the present partly by being compared to a past that differs from it. Anthropology offers a transcultural rather than transtemporal comparison, but there are similarities in the benefits to be gained as well as in the obvious intellectual and psychological efforts of transposing oneself from the familiar and apparently self-evident to the unfamiliar, where meaningfulness must be discovered rather than assumed.

There is a similar connection, of course, between most any historical subject and its counterpart in anthropology.[15] But there were other links of a specifically medical nature. For instance, medical anthropology has a tendency to focus on the act of healing. Indeed, it has been said that anthropology typically studies medicine from the point of view of patients and their families whereas sociology (and, one might add, much social history of medicine) is more interested in the physician and his institutions.[16] Whatever the truth of this, there certainly was a strong orientation, in the anthropology with which I became acquainted, to what goes on in practice. This struck me as a salutary corrective to medical historiography's heavy emphasis on the nonclinical. And talk of "healers" comes to the heart of the matter without being overly selective on the basis of the qualifications and legitimacy of those who are doing the healing.

Obviously one doesn't need anthropology to focus attention on the healing act. Some of our colleagues have been calling for such an approach for years and many social historians of medicine today are addressing this subject, presumably without any special indebtedness to that sister discipline.[17] Nevertheless, anthropology is an avenue to this perspective and has its own particular insights to offer. At any rate, that was the particular road that I took.

Another dimension was offered by the particular type of anthropology to which I was first exposed; namely, cognitive and ethnographic studies. Among other things, they spoke of "belief systems" to refer to the body of thought which lies behind indigenous practices. Such talk of "beliefs" was a refreshing reminder that the healer's corpus of "knowledge" was culturally contingent. This struck me as a welcome emphasis in the face of our tendency to think of our medicine as based on non-culture-bound (timeless, ahistoric) "truths." We need not necessarily believe that all our science is culturally contingent to appreciate the heuristic value of treating at least some of it as if it were.[18] In medicine, in particular, such an approach is surely warranted when the role of science in the healing art is, to say the least, problematical.

But there was an even more fundamental appeal. Cognitive anthropology concerns itself with what people think and how they explain their own behavior, and it gathers evidence for this by consulting particular individuals, the chief actors in the behavior it is trying to understand. It gives credence and significance to the values and concepts of its informants, granting them a causal relationship in the cultural events being witnessed.

The result of such an approach struck me as being at once both social and humanistic: social because the behavior of large groups was being explained; humanistic because account was taken of an individual reality which, however different from ours, was expressed in human terms and on a human scale to which we can relate out of the concreteness of our own personal experience.

This contrasts with the abstract world of much social science that deals with the reality of the aggregate, of the collectivity, and that seeks to uncover the larger, unconscious, unarticulated forces behind the reasons people offer for their behavior. One does not have to doubt the validity of these more comprehensive accounts of human society to feel estranged from them, to feel a lack of their immediacy and relevance in the affairs of the individual. It is simply not the way we personally experience our lives, and the evidence adduced in support of the machinations of large-scale forces, being largely statistical and probabilistic, lacks cogency when reductively applied to individuals, and is downright suspect when applied to the particular individuals whom we encounter in our lives or in the historical record.[19]

In this sense, anthropology appeared to me as an important mediator between the scientific and the cultural, between the social and the intellectual, and between the collective and the individual or, as I think of it, between the social science and the humanistic study of humankind.

The impact of anthropology on medical history can also be substantive. It offers fresh motivation for acquiring a greater knowledge of the world's great traditional systems of medicine, for becoming interested in healers unorthodox as well as orthodox, and for seeing cultural contexts as richly instructive rather than scientifically irrelevant. And it offers frameworks for analysis and for the organization of historical material that really do engage student interest, and that do diminish cultural as well as temporal parochialism.

It was not that anthropology revolutionized or overturned my conventional notions of medical historiography. Rather, it introduced a freshness that has been stimulating. Galenism, taught as a traditional medicine, to be compared with other traditional systems, has been suggestive of new questions and perhaps new insights. Medical astrology in the Renaissance, seen through the eyes of anthropology, seems to me to receive its proper cultural accreditation in a way that had not been achieved by history alone.[20]

All of which is not to say that other social sciences had no part in the evolution of medical-history teaching at McGill. On the contrary, the social events in the Quebec of that period, already described, and the intellectual ambiance that they created, were much more related to areas that are the traditional domain of sociology—medical institutions, education, economics, and professionalization. It was also at this time that collaboration began with Joseph Lella, who had been teaching medical sociology to our medical students since 1965, and who, upon appointment to the department in 1973, became the first to represent us in a field other than history.

Of greatest impact on my own thinking, relative to the teaching of medical history, was the burgeoning literature on medical professionalism.[21] This seemed particularly worthwhile for two reasons. First, it offered a highly useful theme for the organization of much information about physicians, particularly concerning events in the modern period. Second, it struck me that, with its perspectives, a contribution could be made to the student's growing sense of his or her own professional identity.[22] This in turn has been consistent with the department's growing conviction, over the years, that one of our primary responsibilities is to prepare medical students for the rapid changes going on in the social context of medical practice. The social history of medicine and the sociology which it can make use of are thus directly serviceable in the education of tomorrow's physician. It is no accident, then, that the most recent full-time colleague to join us, George Weisz, is a social historian and sociologist.

Not all the valuable large-scale perspectives on medicine have come from sociology, of course. Much fertile ground for survey course or seminar has been opened up by historical demography and by the perspectives of a René Dubos, a Thomas McKeown, or a William McNeill. And what a delightful and stimulating contribution Alfred Crosby's *The Columbian Exchange* has been![23] Perhaps the rarefied Foucault and the prophetlike Illich are not the stuff of general surveys but they make marvellous challenges for intensive seminars or especially interested students, as well as provoking us, as teachers, to uncover the assumptions and biases articulated in the unseen skeletons of our own historical constructions.[24]

Our survey course is still evolving, but these are some of the reasons for the trends it has followed. How much it still owes to that history of public health course, inherited over fifteen years ago from Dr. Temkin, is hard to tell, but it is a lot. His was a good course and it has been built upon and adapted, not replaced.

I want to turn now from content to style and organization. This too owes something to Dr. Temkin's lectures, but, in this case, his survey course to medical students. In that course, Dr. Temkin designed each lecture differently, that is to say with different emphases designed to reflect different historical periods. He constructed his lecture on Arabic medicine, for example, around many anecdotes, ending with the observation that Arabic medicine was often taught in anecdotal form! His lecture on Vesalian anatomy was rich with illustrations of Renaissance art. In doing such things, he was well aware that he was simultaneously satisfying a variety of students' likes and interests. The medical students of McGill enjoy that stylistic variety as much in 1981 as the Hopkins students did twenty years ago.

A second feature follows from the first. No lecture is merely an arbitrary slice of the whole, but an individually designed piece meant to stand more or less on its own. Ninety-minute lectures have made this easier. These individual units are strung upon threads of thematic material that tie them together in some unified, if not always continuous, whole.

Some threads extend only a short distance, but two themes in particular intertwine from beginning to end. These are the intellectual, social, and cultural history of the healer, on the one hand, and the natural history of health and disease in populations, on the other. The two are handled as separate, and largely independent, strands and the course is stitched together with discontinuous and discrete segments of each.

That the health and diseases of populations has a history, that the healer, in his science, practice, education, institutions, and social position likewise has a history, and that neither the present disease situation, nor the social context of the physician is static, nor likely to remain so even during the student's lifetime, seem worthwhile messages, lessons which only history can teach. That the two have proceeded largely in response to quite separate forces, and that their interconnection is problematical and itself the subject of changing attitudes over time, seem even more worthwhile points to make to people beginning the study of medicine.

Apart from comments about content and organization, some observations might be made about the more practical and technical aspects of teaching the course. Evaluations by students, in the form of questionnaires, were conducted for a number of years, and these provided some information of a statistical sort. Discussions during class time and comments after class were another basis for impressions. But most of all, my decision not to have an examination and not to enforce attendance at lectures, even though it is a "required" course in the core curriculum, meant that there was some (but only some) relation between student receptivity of the material and the numbers who faithfully attended lectures. Fifteen years of experience with this approach have led me to certain conclusions about what will encourage or discourage medical student attendance when they have the choice.[25]

First, I believe that the content and skill in delivery of the material is more potent as a negative effect on attendance than as a positive one. Bad teaching, of itself, will rapidly diminish numbers, if students are free not to attend; the attractive effects of good teaching, on the other hand, can, with dismaying ease, be offset by external factors: a medical faculty's lack of symbolic commitment to the subject; poor timing of lectures in the week, or in the day, or in relation to other courses; the pressure of other studies, exams, and the like. At McGill, conditions are optimal: the provision of core-curriculum time; late Monday- and Friday-morning scheduling, preceded and followed by other non-basic-science courses; and course termination before the first serious set of tests.

Second, insofar as the course design itself has an influence, the skillful presentation of pertinent visual material ranks among the top factors in maintaining student interest and thereby attendance. In my experience, the building of a good slide collection has taken years and is still going on, because it is a very personal thing involving modalities of taste and interest that are not governed solely by the historical record.

In terms of lecturing style, the most successful in this subject, as in most others to large classes, I suspect, involves four ingredients: the radiation of personal energy; the projection of a distinctive personality (the type is less important); a largely understated but thoroughly convincing grasp of one's subject matter; and a strong and visible conviction on the part of the lecturer that the subject is interesting and worthwhile.

Enthusiasm for a new course is usually infectious and usually contributes substantially to short-term success. I have never trusted published accounts of how to go about teaching something which are based on one or two years of experience. A course matures, evolves, and takes on richer meaning when taught for several years, especially if it is a survey. If it is a very narrow topic, and especially if it is a topic that is currently in vogue, interest palls—certainly after five years, frequently after three.

Only as a distant third would I put the course content itself, so far as student receptivity is concerned. There are two reasons for this. The first is that, as already explained, tailoring course content to impressions of prevailing classroom interests may, in reality, be appealing only to the interests of a dominant few. This will have no appreciable effect on attendance, which is affected by the particular outlooks and interests of each and every individual. And if one seeks to relate course material to those underlying preferences, such differing and sometimes conflicting tastes and views exist as to make a unanimous or even widespread student consensus difficult, if not impossible, to find. If the sole criterion of course content were student receptivity as reflected in attendance, the best approach would most likely be a great men, great ideas, great events approach, provided, of course, that the external factors mentioned earlier did not work against it. But this is only a guess because I have never granted class attendance such an overriding priority as to resort to something which I believe would be an inadequate discharge of one's academic responsibilities.

The second reason why I think student receptivity is a lesser guide for deciding on course content (although I would not dismiss it altogether by any means) has to do with prevailing attitudes about history, generally. In North America at least, the dominant values in medicine, reflected by the profession, by medical institutions, by much of the mass media, and by the educational background and the social middle class from which the students come, do not lead students to conclude that a historical perspective—any historical perspective on any subject matter—is as valuable to becoming a doctor as is anatomy, or biochem-

istry, or pathology. The basic sciences are taken as self-evidently relevant. The basis for such self-evidence comes not simply from their
demonstrable effects on medical practice, but from their share of the
symbol and value placed upon science in medicine in our present society. Hence the teaching of these subjects, even when poor, irrelevant,
uninteresting, or burdensome, can still command faculty support and
student attention without being required to justify itself. But medical
history is not in that position and no amount of philosophizing about,
or tinkering with, the course content is going to cure the subject of its
shaky status in the medical system of values.

For the better part of this century, medical history, taught inside
medical centers or outside of them, has been problematical for the simple reason that modern medicine itself has *not* been problematical for
the great majority of people. Freed from temporal and social contingency, the only thing that the recently uncovered, timeless truths of this
new medicine seemed to need was people to celebrate the story of their
discovery and to be custodians of their genealogy.

Fortunately, things are changing. Today, no serious student of the
phenomenon called "modern medicine," now global in its distribution
and impact, is any longer content with the parochial perspective of a
single society. As we watch this medicine diffuse into other societies
and confront other medicines, the case for seeing it once again as itself a
historical and cultural product becomes impossible to avoid. Just what
is this thing called "science" that Western society has developed? What
role has it played in the healing art, or in providing for the health of
populations? Is there a limit to its application? Have we reached or
exceeded that limit? What about industrialization, with its attendant
urbanization, affluence, and technological conversion of materials and
values? How have these shaped the medicine we have, or, for that matter, the problems that our medicine is intended to solve? How did what
we have now evolve from our own prescientific, preindustrial past?
What connection does that premodern medicine have with the indigenous medicines of other cultures that are now extant?

The questions, and the possibilities for historical research, are
endless. Medicine today needs all the historical perspective—intellectual (most particularly including the history of its sciences), social, and
natural—that we can furnish. If we fail to convey that fact to our
medical colleagues or to our medical students, it may be, paradoxically,
because they or we are not yet up to date. It does seem, at any rate, that
an appreciation of the past requires a firm grasp of the present.

It will be clear by now that the evolution of our course has been the
outcome of many influences: the local conditions of tradition and support that provided baseline institutional security; the background, pro-
clivities, and problems of the individual designing and giving the

course; the changing social context and its impact on the outlook of all concerned; the special developments of the social sciences and growing involvement with them; and the vicissitudes of a classroom situation where attendance was open both to the internal influence of course content and teaching skills and to the external pressures of other courses and alternative values.

What has been the outcome? It is difficult to say. A personal impression is that the course has continuing, possibly increasing, credibility among the students and medical faculty. Certainly there is considerable evidence that it has become a contributing part of our broader, departmental program aimed at challenging students to widen their horizons, to discover and to review their assumptions and values, to achieve growth and sophistication in their personal and professional identities, and to acquire a sense of the temporal and cultural relatedness of the careers for which they are preparing.[26]

The result for me personally is that early misgivings have been dispelled, and I have come to feel strongly that such a course is worthwhile and that the larger program of which it is a part is essential. Indeed, I would go so far as to claim that fulfillment of the aims of the program, mentioned above, should be as obligatory a part of medical education as are physiology and internal medicine.

At the same time, it should be pointed out that our survey course in the history of medicine is just that. It is not a course in humanities; it is not co-taught with people from other disciplines.[27] What it has gained from other fields of study have been fresh suggestions as to appropriate subject matter, promising lines of analysis, and additional reasons for being taught. But it remains a course in history and we see no reason to change that. Moreover, it is a broad survey which reaches back to the earliest historic times and we see no reason to change that either.

Are there any general conclusions to be drawn from this McGill experience? My own inclination is to say that any qualified person who has the chance to teach medical history to medical students should do so, should offer a course that is unapologetic and unadulterated history, and should make it as unrestricted in time span, variety of subject matter, and geography as opportunity permits. Such an effort should obviously be coupled with the motivation to do a good job, and, no less obviously perhaps, with modest expectations as to the result. But those modest expectations should not be an excuse for not doing it, nor for not trying to do it well.

However, the only generalization to which I am fully committed is that the best teaching is tailored to a particular professor, to specific students, and to the local situation. That is because, for me, teaching, like healing, is a humanistic, not a scientific undertaking.[28] It was in this spirit, as the practitioner of a craft, that I have chosen the risky

stratagem of autobiography. If I have offended, I plead my case with the
dictum of Carl Rogers: "What is most personal is most general." [29]

Notes

1. John B. Blake, ed., *Education in the History of Medicine: Report of a Macy Conference Sponsored by the Josiah Macy, Jr., Foundation in Cooperation with the National Library of Medicine, Bethesda, Maryland, June 22–24, 1966* (New York: Hafner Publishing, 1968).

2. "The history of medicine as a part of the university complex," ibid., pp. 85–92.

3. See *The Osler Library*, McGill University, published on the occasion of the fiftieth anniversary of the library in 1979.

4. For example, the Osler Library is governed by a board of curators created by Sir William Osler's instructions, which provided that the principal of the university and the dean of medicine be *ex officio* members, the latter as board chairman. See Nancy Grant, "Sir William and the Osler Library's board of curators," *Osler Library Newsletter,* No. 2 (1969). The *Newsletter,* begun in 1969, and the Friends of the Osler Library, started in 1972, further strengthened this tradition.

5. Each year, one lecture of the survey course, to be described below, is devoted to the history of the McGill Medical Faculty and is one of the most popular among our medical students. The lecture is given by E. H. Bensley, for many years a professor of medicine and historian of the faculty, now emeritus professor and, since 1968, a part-time member of our department.

6. See Lloyd G. Stevenson, "The translation of the Osler Library from the Strathcona Building to the McIntyre Building," *Osler Library Newsletter* 14 (1973).

7. At the time, however, this view was defended on political grounds. A report to the Wellcome Trust, 26 February 1970, states, "In the present context in which the Department finds itself, it is not reasonable to request the continued addition of specifically medical historians to be supported by the Medical Faculty when the contribution of each additional member would mean, at best, five to ten percent involvement in Medical Faculty educational activities." As a solution it was contemplated that the department would broaden its subject matter to include "the social sciences in medicine" and/or "the history of the life sciences." Among the social sciences, sociology, anthropology, and economics were offered as possible examples.

8. A letter to the Wellcome Trust, of 20 May 1971, reports that "over the course of this year, this Department floated the idea of [expansion which] . . . might be reflected in some such title as the 'Department of Social and Humanities Studies in Medicine.'" The actual change of name to "Department of Humanities and Social Studies in Medicine" was approved by McGill's board of governors in December 1980, long after the department had, in fact, widened its scope.

9. See Charles Webster, "Medicine as social history: changing ideas on doctors and patients in the age of Shakespeare," in *A Celebration of Medical History,* ed. Lloyd G. Stevenson (Baltimore: The Johns Hopkins University Press, 1982), for a discussion of British medical historiography during the twentieth century, and my "Commentary" on Webster's paper for a discussion of North American historiography, where the subject of the influence of the history of science, among other influences, is enlarged upon.

10. This impression is based on as yet unpublished statistics that we have accumulated on the five most recent classes of second-year medical students concerning their attitudes to social issues related to health care.

11. For a highly readable account of these remarkable events, see Malcolm Taylor, *Health Insurance and Canadian Public Policy: The Seven Decisions that Created the Canadian Health Insurance System,* Institute of Public Administration of Canada (Montreal: McGill-Queens Press, 1978), pp. 379–413.

12. Sidney S. Lee has written a succinct summary (fifty-four pages) of this evolution, *Quebec's Health System: A Decade of Change, 1967–77,* Monographs on Canadian Public Administration, No. 4, Institute of Public Administration of Canada (n.p., 1979).

13. The department does other medical history teaching to medical students individually, in electives, and in groups of eight to twelve in a seminar for final-year students, but this paper will concentrate on the survey course taught to all medical students in the first year of a four-year M.D. program.

14. See John M. Janzen, *The Quest for Therapy in Lower Zaire* (Berkeley: University of California Press, 1978) for the final fruit of his research.

15. I have long been an admirer of E. R. Dodds's use of anthropology and psychology in *The Greeks and the Irrational* (1951; reprint ed., Berkeley: University of California Press, 1968) and, more recently, of Keith Thomas's *Religion and the Decline of Magic: Studies in Popular Beliefs in Sixteenth- and Seventeenth-Century England* (Hammondsworth, Middlesex, England: Penguin

Books, 1971). For a review of this latter work and an expression of qualified dissent, see E. P. Thompson, "Anthropology and the discipline of historical context," *Midland History,* 1971, *1:* 41–55.

16. See, for example, George M. Foster, "Medical anthropology: some contrasts with medical sociology," *Medical Anthropology Newsletter* 6, no. 1 (1974). Included in the same issue is "Convergences and divergences: anthropology and sociology in health care," by Virginia L. Olesen.

17. A recent example is Charles Webster, "Medicine as social history," n. 9, above.

18. For a demonstration of this approach to biology see Barry Barnes and Steve Shapin, eds., *Natural Order: Historical Studies of Scientific Culture,* (Beverly Hills: Sage Publications, 1979). A fairly closely argued and brief critique of the recent thoughts of historians of science and sociologists on the social contingency of scientific knowledge is offered by Michael Mulkay, *Science and the Sociology of Knowledge* (London: George Allen & Unwin, 1979).

19. Despite difficulties, the department is convinced that the insights of the social sciences are important for medical students, as will be seen below. In order to give these insights more personal meaning, however, an individualistic or humanistic orientation is applied to them when possible. We have come to speak of such adaptations as "social studies," hence the use of this term in the department's new name. For an appeal to integrate "micro-analysis" with "macro-analysis" in the study of medical systems, see John Janzen, "The comparative study of medical systems as changing social systems," *Social Science and Medicine,* 1978, *12:* 121–29.

20. I am thinking here of Keith Thomas's chapter on astrology in his *Religion and the Decline of Magic.*

21. Although his historical introduction leaves something to be desired, and not everyone would agree with his treatment of scientific knowledge in medical practice, Eliot Freidson's *Profession of Medicine: A Study of the Sociology of Applied Knowledge* (New York: Dodd, Mead, & Co., 1971) was a landmark study on its appearance a decade ago.

22. See Joseph W. Lella, "Les sciences sociales et la formation du medecin: vers une pédagogie de l'identité médicale," *Le médecin du Québec,* 1980, *15:* 117–41, for a more comprehensive formulation of this objective. Dr. Lella and I have worked so closely together for the past eight years that many of the ideas that I am employing in the present account are the result of our combined experiences and many discussions, and I no longer know who was originally responsible for which.

23. René Dubos, *Mirage of Health: Utopias, Progress, and Biological Change* (London: George Allen & Unwin, 1959); Thomas McKeown, *The Role of Medicine: Dream, Mirage, or Nemesis?* (London: The Nuffield Provincial Hospitals Trust, 1976); William H. McNeill, *Plagues and Peoples* (New York: Anchor Press, 1976); Alfred W. Crosby, Jr., *The Columbian Exchange: The Biological and Cultural Consequences of 1492* (Westport, Conn.: Greenwood Press, 1972).

24. For each of the past five years, the department has taught an intensive, one-month seminar to eight to twelve final-year students called "Illich and His Critics." Besides Dubos and McKeown, mentioned above, the students discuss several of the works of Ivan Illich, including *Limits to Medicine: Medical Nemesis, the Expropriation of Health* (London: McClelland & Stewart, 1976), as well as Vincente Navarro, *Medicine under Capitalism* (New York: Prodist, 1976), and several other works. History is a major, working component in all of these critiques of present-day medicine.

25. Over the years, many "head counts," from the back of the lecture hall, have been done. The patterns of attendance have varied for individual lectures but the trend over the duration of the course has remained quite stable from year to year. There is a more or less slow but steady attrition. Attendance at the final lecture has been as low as 30 students, more typically 40 to 50, in the most recent year, 85. Class size began at 135 but has been 160 for many years. A meaningful examination for that many students, to be marked by one individual, has always been difficult to conceive. Moreover, no appropriate textbook to complement the course has been found.

26. In another course on the social aspects of current medicine, emphasis is on Canada and particularly on Quebec. This is all the more reason for a history course to range widely in time and space.

27. The department does teach collaborative, nondisciplinary courses in the medical core curriculum in "Behavior" (which deals with the psychological and social experience of health and illness and with the implications of these for the practicing physician), in "The Physician and Society," and in "Medical Ethics and Jurisprudence." Our staff also teaches disciplinary courses in medical anthropology, medical sociology, and medical history within the respective departments of the arts faculty. Unfortunately, for largely technical reasons, only a small percentage of entering medical students have been previously exposed to these arts courses.

28. An attitude explained at greater length in "Humanism in undergraduate medical education," *Canad. Med. Assoc. J.,* 1971, *105:* 258–61.

29. Carl R. Rogers, *On Becoming a Person* (Boston: Houghton Mifflin, 1961), p. 26.

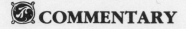

COMMENTARY

Lloyd G. Stevenson

As Professor Bates has pointed out in a note, his paper was not presented at the symposium; because, however, of the unusual nature of his department—its recent change of name represents the development over fifteen years of a surprisingly comprehensive entity— it was thought desirable to include his story with the others. It is the interesting story of the growth of a department and, concurrently, of the evolution of a course, but although "a fairly personal account of the events at McGill's medical school," it is related fairly closely to developments in other centers—in medical history as social history, as medical sociology, and as medical anthropology. Others taking part in the symposium have shown a somewhat similar inclination to "broaden the disciplinary base," but its breadth and solidity seem to be particularly well attested in Don G. Bates's paper. Despite the autobiographical character of the narrative ("What is most personal is most general" reads the paradox of Carl Rogers) it shows "the changing social context and its impact on the outlook of all concerned." The changing social context referred to is, essentially, although not exclusively, the novel health care system of Quebec. In this, of course, the narrative is not paralleled, at least not in the same way, and so the tale is both a general one and a particular one.

McGill was characterized, at Bates's beginning, by "exceptional institutional supports." The Osler Library, the Osler-Francis tradition, and new physical facilities were all unusual. "Most important, there was a strong tradition of interest in the history of medicine that had already existed for almost half a century." Osler, then, stood in the background, a little dimly but nevertheless distinctly present. In the foreground there were, at any rate, splendid physical facilities. One has the impression of an echoing, empty palace—which is the way in which a good story now and again begins. It was in order to "end isolation" that measures were taken to reach out from mere medical history to a wide range of humanities and social sciences. Initially this appeared, or so in retrospect it seems, to have been something of almost desperate urgency, expansion being seen as "virtually impossible" without it; it was later perceived that "the department might have been granted some growth strictly within the confines of medical history." The outreach program had, however, begun—and there is no questioning the tremendous zeal and the palpable success which have marked its career.

It is an interesting coincidence that the Institute of the History of Medicine at the Johns Hopkins University and the Osler Library at McGill University were opened for business in the same year, the one centering on William H. Welch, the other on William Osler. Harvey Cushing, Osler's biographer, and John F. Fulton, Cushing's biographer, initiated, with the help of Arnold Klebs, the great Historical Library at Yale, and also the Department of the History of Science and Medicine—which, although it subsequently foundered, has been gloriously reborn in the area where it first began, in the history of medicine. Is this the only way in which such a program can be launched and maintained? Does it require the energy, the charisma, the determination—and also the books—of some glittering hero, or more than one, before it can be established? Must these be included as necessary among "exceptional institutional supports?" Not all of the centers represented in this symposium quite fit that pattern. It is interesting, however, to observe and to compare. When Bates tells us of the tentative association, at McGill, between the history of medicine and the history of science—an association that somehow failed to work out—we are reminded of the ambition of Richard H. Shryock, an ambition never achieved, to expand Welch's Institute in Baltimore to encompass the history of science; instead of this, Johns Hopkins established History of Science as a friendly but quite distinct department. Are the history of medicine and the history of science for some reason incompatible? Such a generalization would be difficult indeed to uphold, even though Harvard, with its superb libraries and manifold resources, has not succeeded, thus far, in welding the history of science and the history of medicine together in any really impressive fashion.

It is not, of course, departmental structure alone that Don Bates has discussed. The recent change of his department's name, in fact, has been adopted to correspond to its achieved identity. The course, rather than (or prior to) the department—has evolved in the direction of the broadly conceived medical humanities and social sciences. At the same time, although sharing in the now common conviction that "the historiography of medicine . . . has been unduly oriented to the history of medical sciences," Bates has conceded that "the [McGill] commitment to social history was not wholehearted, or perhaps I should say, not comprehensive." He has not, in other words, cast aside the history of the medical sciences. His admirable aim has been to omit no promising approach.

Bates has told the story, or a part of the story, of medical history at

McGill, and has not aimed at a more general account of the development of medical-history teaching. Perhaps it need not be pointed out, then, that more than thirty years ago a medical historian who also enjoys a distinguished reputation as anthropologist—Erwin H. Ackerknecht—was teaching in Madison, Wisconsin, a course that might easily have been labeled "Humanities and Social Sciences in Medicine," nor that Owsei Temkin taught for many years in Baltimore a program as close to total history (and *histoire totale* has of course never excluded the humanities and social sciences) as has ever been attempted in any medical school anywhere. To both of these assertions Don Bates would be happy, I think, to assent, and he would doubtless agree, also, that all modern medical historians can trace some part of their expanded awareness of the medical humanities and social sciences to Henry Sigerist's Leipzig Institute around about 1930.

And yet such a course as the one here described for McGill—a course developed from personal sources of inspiration—has been and remains a rarity to be cherished and emulated.

STARTING FROM SCRATCH: INSTALLING A HISTORY OF MEDICINE PROGRAM IN A NEW MEDICAL SCHOOL

Robert J. T. Joy

This essay describes how the teaching of medical history was introduced in a new medical school in 1976 and how the program developed over the next five years.

The law founding the Uniformed Services University of the Health Sciences provides for only one statutory faculty member, "a professor of military, naval or air science." This was interpreted by the board of regents and the dean to require a professor and a Department of Military Medicine. Since no American medical school had ever had such a department (for obvious reasons) the scope for curriculum planning was both unknown and open-ended.

In the discussions that led to my appointment as department chairman, I expressed my strong conviction that the history of medicine, with an emphasis on military medical history, should be an integral part of the curriculum of the department and the school. The dean, Jay Sanford, was enthusiastic. Not only did he have a personal interest in medical history, but he believed that in a new school without its own traditions learning about the work and contributions of military medicine and medical officers would provide the medical students with a sense of community and connection with the past. To emphasize this, the new department was named the Department of Military Medicine and History.

The medical faculty were and are extraordinarily supportive. With the exception of two medical officers, the original faculty of 1976–1977 (who designed the curriculum of the first two years) were all distinguished civilian teachers from other medical schools. Not a single civilian department chairman came from a school that had a medical history course; yet, without exception, they were enthusiastic about having one and posed no problems in assigning curriculum hours. Several of them have audited the course.

When curriculum planning for the school began in 1976, the history of medicine was allocated thirty-four lecture hours in the freshman year. My basic assumptions about curriculum content were laid down that first year and have not changed very much. The focus of the course would be on European and American medical history. We would not teach Indian, Chinese, or Japanese medical history. This decision was made in part because of lack of personal expertise and difficulty in securing visiting lecturers on these topics, and in part because these cultures have not been major contributors to the general development of Western medicine. The course would give a chronological review of European and American medical history as a survey course. We must remember that all basic-science courses in medical schools are survey courses. The emphasis within the course would be on what is called "internal" or "iatrocentric" history, although there would be lectures that emphasized the "external" history of medicine in its larger social, institutional, and cultural aspects.

I believe that medicine is and will remain eponymal. How sad to hold a Kelly clamp, feel a Corrigan pulse, do a Halsted repair, see a patient with Addison's disease—and have no knowledge of who these physicians were or how they lived and worked. Thus, there was to be discussion of the great men and women. Without playing "hip, hip, Hippocrates," and with attempts to show them warts and all, I proceeded in the belief that the students should know most of the major and some of the secondary people in medicine.

In short, I wanted the curriculum to show how—by fits and starts and with many false trails—medicine grew from magic and religion and slowly arrived at the state of the art the students find today. I believe that medical students will best respond to being taught medical history if they can see some connection to what they are learning in other courses and if they can grasp the relationship between the practice of the past and the practice they are entering. But I interpret "practice" broadly, to include the interactions between the larger society and the institutions of medicine.

I outlined a series of thirty-four lectures intended to show the students where physicians came from, how medical education developed, how medical practice moved from the library to the bedside to the hospital to the laboratory, and how the hospital developed as the doctor's workplace. They were to hear how science entered medicine, how medicine organized itself as a profession, how medicine began in America from its European roots, and how the medical problems of people and populations gradually changed—in the West—from epidemic infectious diseases to chronic diseases. Topics on military medical history were interspersed at the appropriate chronological points. The themes of these latter lectures were the slow evolution of the position and function of the physician on the battlefield and at sea, and the special problems—surgical, disease, evacuation, hospitalization—of military medicine, their recognition and solution.

The course outline was then discussed with several senior historians of medicine, all of whom are still active in teaching. They made extraordinarily valuable suggestions for topic area, specific approach, and course integration. It was obvious that I had neither the competence nor the time to deliver thirty-four lectures in such a survey course. I turned to colleagues in the history of medicine at universities, medical schools, and the National Library of Medicine, and asked if they would help by giving a one-hour general lecture in the field of their expertise. Obviously, I asked teachers whose area of interest matched the topics chosen for the course. Without exception, they all responded magnificently, often at some inconvenience to themselves in the arranging of their schedules. In the beginning, nineteen of the thirty-four lectures were given by visiting colleagues and fifteen by myself. As my views of the course developed and changed, and given time over the years to prepare my own lectures on certain topics, this has now been reduced to twelve visiting teachers for forty-three lectures. The present list of medical-student lectures is attached as an appendix.

With rare exceptions, all courses at our school are graded, and the medical-history course is no exception. It is a two-credit course and the grade is based upon a twelve-to-fifteen-page original paper on any topic the student chooses. I require the students to discuss their topic with me before they begin. This protects them from choosing too grandiose a theme and, for those who have trouble selecting a topic, allows me to explore their interests, and guide them to one. Each of these interviews lasts thirty to forty minutes, allowing me to discuss how one finds sources, frames a paper, organizes the writing, handles references, and so on. This is time-consuming, but it provides the only opportunity for one-on-one teaching in the history course. The Washington area is rich in specialty libraries in addition to the Library of Congress, the National Library of Medicine, and the other great collections in Washington. Our university librarians are superb at arranging for the students to use or borrow from these splendid collections, and this extends the opportunities for the students to use primary source material whenever appropriate.

The formal requirements for the paper, along with general guidelines, are handed out in September; the paper is due in early June. I read all papers and use the same general criteria I use in refereeing manuscripts for journals. Their grade depends—as the guidelines have told them—on organization of their discussion, originality of approach, evidence of logical thought, proper use of sources, and a clear writing style, as well as on grammar, syntax, and spelling. It takes about an hour to read, comment on, and grade each paper. As I consider this my last chance to teach in the course, I write extensive comments on each paper, complimentary or critical, so that the students, in reading the returned papers, will have had one final chance at a dialogue.

In 1978 the faculty, agreeing that our initial curriculum was too dense, introduced examination weeks and decreased teaching hours by about 10 percent. The result of these changes was to decrease the history course from thirty-four to thirty-three hours. At this time, the chairman of the Department of Preventive Medicine offered me three hours in his curriculum to give certain lectures in the history of epidemiology and infectious diseases. In my own curriculum in military medicine I had decided that the introductory lectures to current issues in military medicine would best be done if given as historical lectures. As the school established a sophomore course in medical ethics it seemed appropriate to have two of the thirty-six hours of that course devoted to history. The net result of these changes was to increase the hours for history of medicine to forty-three hours in the first two years.

As mentioned previously, many of the faculty audited the medical-student course, attending certain of the lectures because of an interest in the topic. As a result, there have been requests that historical seminars be given to their own department's graduate students. We now do this three or four times a year in various departments and plan to expand this participation in the graduate programs as invited and as feasible.

By 1978 I believed I was ready for the next phase of the history program: continuing medical education (CME) and house officer teaching. The military medical special schools and hospitals have the same requirements for CME accreditation and licensure that civilian institutions do. Using an "old boy network," I offered a selected list of lecture topics to such institutions as the Army Academy of Health Sciences and the Air Force School of Aerospace Medicine. These relationships have now grown to eighteen lectures a year, given to various of their postgraduate courses in military medicine, preventive medicine, aerospace medicine, and so on.

As "the word" spread about the availability of history lectures, and particularly lectures on the history of military medicine, invitations began to arrive from military and civilian hospitals. At this writing, I average ten lectures a year, all over the country. These audiences may be house staff, attending staff, or—in the case of several civilian institutions—practicing private physicians. I am convinced there is an eager audience among house staff and practicing physicians for lectures in the history of medicine. These groups are perfectly content to hear a lecture on nearly any topic, but they prefer material on medically oriented history as I have described it above.

Again through personal friendships, I began in 1979 to lecture to the pediatric house staff at Walter Reed Army Medical Center during their weekly grand-rounds conferences. This has now grown to eight scheduled lectures a year, and this year (1981) it has been expanded to the pediatric combined staff conference at the National Naval Medical Center, where we are still exploring the number and content of the lectures to be given.

The final outreach program was to the military history community, with which I have had a long affiliation. Due to the fact that each of the services has a military- or naval-history organization to produce its official histories and direct its museums, and to the presence of the National Archives, the Library of Congress, and the National Library of Medicine, Washington has a large number of historians who work for the federal government. Personal contact and the offering of topics in military medical history have made it possible for me to give three or four seminars a year to various of these groups. This has also provided invaluable access to military-history experts and sources critical to my own research interests.

Finally, as an experiment, next year the introductory lecture in the Department of Anatomy will be on the history of anatomy. If this is successful, I will approach other department chairmen, in both basic and clinical sciences, and explore the possibility of doing this in each of their courses. If they can be persuaded to this, then—as is now done in the Department of Preventive Medicine—lectures can be moved from the freshman course in medical history and those hours used to expand the core curriculum in history. I plan to use these hours to introduce more social history of medicine in the course. Another approach will be to build on the success of a two-hour seminar in an advanced senior medical-student elective in medical ethics and offer single seminars on the historical background of the topics of other senior elected courses.

In summary, then: at the medical school and to outside audiences, I am able to provide about forty-five teaching hours of medical history to medical students and about forty to forty-five hours to other medical and historical groups.

The program must be placed in perspective. The department has 190 teaching hours in the freshman and sophomore years; of these the medical history course has 33 hours, the rest are devoted to modern military medicine. The department also directs four four-week orientation courses for freshmen in service-specific basic officer training. The department faculty are responsible for a five-week course in field applications of military medicine, which is given in the summer between freshman and sophomore year. Finally, the members of the department all have additional duty as the Office of Commandant of Students, responsible for student military affairs and discipline, social and athletic events, and specialized military training. These details are included because it should be made clear that the history program has never been more than a modest part of departmental responsibilities and that, as Department Chairman and Commandant of Students, it could not occupy most of my time, since I also had teaching requirements in military medicine and in physiology.

Well—what general case can be made from this detailed discussion of how one program in medical history got started and how it grew? Let me emphasize that this is description, not prescription. Much of what has been done is perhaps unique to beginning with a new school, to having a dean enthusiastic about history, and a faculty totally supportive of the need for teaching the history of medicine. Not one of the methods of reaching students and audiences is new. What may be new is doing all of the various approaches at once. Unquestionably, as I hope I have made clear, personal relationships of years' standing were responsible for the introduction and beginning of many of the outreach programs in CME, in house staff programs within other teaching departments, and in military history programs. Our students, as commissioned officers on salary, have a longer academic day and year than at the average medical school. We have time in the curriculum for courses in medical humanism.

But there may be some general conclusions that could be helpful to medical historians in other schools. First, to shape the core curriculum as a survey course oriented directly to medical students, to what they are doing and to what they hope to become. They are overwhelmed by their basic-science courses and simultaneously impatient to "get on the wards" and "learn medicine." Therefore, a course content that is weighted toward the history of the medical sciences, of medical practice, of disease, and of the "great doctors" is far more likely to capture their interest than a curriculum focused on the social history of medicine. The teacher must assume that the class as a whole knows no history and must therefore integrate general history into the medical topic, or the students will be lost in isolated facts, places, and people and will not know either where or when they are. At our school—and I suspect at others—about 35 percent of our freshmen are biology majors, another 30 percent or so are chemistry majors, and all but 5 to 6 percent of the rest were trained in the physical, social, or engineering sciences. Of those with humanities degrees, only a few were history majors. At our present average class size of 130, I find only 2 or 3 students with history degrees, and—in the premedical majors—never more than 1 or 2 who had an undergraduate course in the history of medicine. As I discuss elsewhere in this volume, illustrated lectures, familiar to students in their basic science courses, are most likely to capture their attention.

I suggest that colleagues in other medical-school departments might be very amenable to including history lectures in their courses, if one is willing to give the lecture *they* want, not the one the historian thinks they should have. This does not mean any loss of professional autonomy or pride—the historian remains in control of the material and the presentation—but we must remember that we are teaching to someone else's curriculum and must be responsive to the overall aim of that schedule.

Outreach programs—to the house staff, to practicing physicians, and to CME programs—take a lot of work, rely heavily on personal relationships, and must also respond to the needs of these programs and their directors. It may seem tedious to trundle across town to the hospital eight times a year to give a historical grand rounds to an audience that is more accustomed to (and may prefer) a discussion of the latest enzyme abnormality. Where is the continuity? Where is the control? Where is the satisfaction of developing one's own students? Well—is it not a teacher's job to teach? If the clinical program directors keep asking you back it's because they—and *their* students—believe they are getting something out of it. Perhaps the real reward is what has now happened to me a half-dozen times since I began teaching house staff; a visit from young residents or fellows who want help in preparing a small historical paper on a topic that interests them or guidance to the history of an area that they have just begun to explore.

The CME programs and the "one-shot" visits to hospitals or medical societies or to groups of other kinds of historians may seem like burdensome diversions from the press of one's own work. And then, one of the physicians who hears you at the medical society CME calls to donate his grandfather's medical books to your library—and the collection includes the original Walter Reed typhoid report!

The writing of this essay in June of 1981 marks a happy change in the medical-history program at the Uniformed Services University of the Health Sciences. In March 1981, the board of regents reviewed the five year development of the program and voted to establish it as an independent Section of Medical History with its own chairman and faculty. The organizational and recruiting plans are underway.* The dean and the faculty have agreed to continue the present teaching programs intact. Further, the Department of Preventive Medicine and Biometrics will establish a Master's of Public Health program in October of 1982 and have asked that a seminar course in the history of public health be established for their students. It appears that the history of medicine has been accepted as an integral and required part of the various curricula of this medical school.

*Note: While this volume was in production, the section was established. Dr. Joy has been selected as chairman, two additional faculty members are being recruited, and the teaching program has expanded to new clinical and basic-science departments.

The theme of this collection of essays is teaching the history of medicine in a medical center. In my view, this means *teaching* first and foremost: teaching the audiences who are assigned to us or whom we recruit; teaching at all levels, from student to house staff to practicing physicians; teaching the fascinating, odd, marvelous, quirky, and captivating history of one of the world's great professions. For those who do not know the history of their profession may be great technicians— but they will not be professionals.

Appendix A

The following lectures are the medical history core curriculum, given once a week throughout the freshman year.

Medicine and War—An Overview
Magic, Myth and Medicine
The Beginnings of Military Medicine: Egypt
Medicine in Greece
Roman Medicine, Empire and Army
History of Anatomy
Development of Military Surgery in the Medieval Period
*Medicine in the Seventeenth and Eighteenth Centuries
*American Medicine in the Colonial Period
*History of Physiology
Military Medicine in the American Revolution
*Epidemic Diseases in America in the Eighteenth and Nineteenth Centuries
*American Clinical Medicine and Sanitary Reform
Military Medicine in the Napoleonic Wars
Naval Medicine: The Age of Fighting Sail
French Clinical Medicine Early in the Nineteenth Century
Henrí Dunant and the Red Cross Movement
The Crimean War and Florence Nightingale
The American Civil War and the Letterman System
*Medicine on the Western Frontier
Microbiology and the Introduction of the Laboratory to Medicine
Military Medical Contributions to Medicine and Science: The People
Military Medical Contributions to Medicine and Science: The Institutions
*Women in Medicine
The History of the U.S. Public Health Service
Naval Medicine in the Steel Navy
*The Development of Modern Psychiatry
*The History of Surgery After Lister
*The History of the Hospital: The Doctor's Workplace
The History of Aviation Medicine
World War I: Modern Medicine in War

*Health Care and the State
World War II: Scientific Medicine in War

Appendix B

The following lectures are given in other courses in preventive medicine, ethics in medicine and military medicine.

Yellow Fever as a Problem in Epidemiology
The Social History of Cholera
Panum on Measles
The Noncombatant Status of Doctor and Patient in War:
    The Geneva Conventions
The Military and Medicine—Ethical Issues
The Responsibilities of the Medical Officer
History of the Organization of the Department of Defense
History of Medical Defense Against Chemical Weapons
The History of the Development of Physical Standards
Cold Injury: Historical and Tactical Implications
Historical Development of Joint Medical Planning and Operations

In addition to these lectures, some of which are given, with modifications to postgraduate medical audiences, I have a "pool" of six to eight other lectures which are more appropriate for these groups.

* Lectures by visiting lecturers.

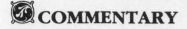# COMMENTARY

Lloyd G. Stevenson

Robert Joy's vigorous account of the inauguration and the first five years of a successful history of medicine program at the Uniformed Services University of the Health Sciences is exhilarating. Has a sparkling, cloudless sky (over Washington?) produced, as it were, an olive drab glow, or is a sort of military medical magic responsible for engendering an especially fruitful climate? Col. Joy concedes that his may well be, in certain obvious respects, a "special case"—of which the most important element, perhaps, is time. "Our students, as commissioned officers on salary, have a longer academic day and year than at the average medical school." And yet, with this and other advantages acknowledged, it is clear that the major elements in the warm reception of the USUHS program have been the basic course and the teachers, or the principal teacher (the Department of Military Medicine and History is also the Office of the Commandant of Students), because their enthusiastic acceptance by staff and by students is plain to be seen. This course, although it claims not to neglect the social, intellectual, and cultural aspects, is frankly iatrocentric in emphasis, an emphasis this discussant, for one, is happy to welcome. Now the "iatrocentric" is considered patently old hat and unacceptable by those historians who have pushed physicians, surgeons, and medical scientists to the periphery of the record. Medical students and doctors are all the same alleged by Joy to be better pleased with this "internal" brand of history. It is nonetheless true that it seems rarely to have pleased many for long, at least when not well interlarded with "external" and even cultural history, as the USUHS course apparently is and as most Johns Hopkins courses have been for many years. Here, of course, there is another factor, not to be counted on elsewhere: more than 45 percent of the basic thirty-three lecture course (how generous an allowance of time in what is universally declared to be the overpacked medical-school curriculum!) is avowedly military. Can the ordinary civilian program benefit in any respect from such an example? If men's (persons') businesses and bosoms are to be reached, possibly the business element, in place of the military, might be somewhat touched upon, or (conversely? concurrently?) health care and the state might receive slightly greater attention. Any number of considerations, cultural and social, might take the place of the ubiquitous military. In any case, this stimulating and still evolving program should be pondered alertly and with care.

It ought not to be assumed by the reader—I think it is not maintained by the author—that the program is, in its essentials, a novel one. The novelty lies in its variety and extent. Its iatrocentric emphasis, although this may yet be rated the minority approach, is in fact the good old standard one, reaching back to the time before the Leipzig Institute as it came to be oriented under Sigerist's direction, and to the time, in America, when medical history, if considered at all, was usually a distillation from Garrison's text. The initiation of another department's course with one or two introductory lectures by a medical historian is a procedure which has been, in many centers, not at all unknown. Neither is the basing of the course grade on a short, original paper, much discussed with the instructor, altogether unexampled.[1] Even the richly illustrated lectures—separately described and exemplified by Col. Joy at a rousing noonday session of this symposium and having, in the manner of their presentation, elements of genuine novelty—are of course not the first attempts of the kind.[2] The request of other disciplines that historical seminars be given to the graduate students of their departments, as well as the "outreach" offerings to house staff, to practicing physicians and to CME programs, make up an impressive array of pedagogical achievements. If the quality of the content, from a professional viewpoint, may be queried—and surely this is permissible in the near absence of professional historical publication not of the how-to-do-it kind—such query would come best, I think, from critics with some more or less comparable claim to teaching success. Of these there are amazingly few.

Whatever the real source of the opinion, there is a saying (supposedly Chinese) that one picture is worth a thousand words. The current counterpart of this is that a thousand pictures leave little need for words at all, although only mathematicians, chemists, and physicists get along handily without them. More than a thousand words, which suffice for the most leisurely commercial, and the effect is considered soporific. About the middle of the last century, William Wordsworth published a rather grumpy sonnet in which he deplored the appearance of illustrated journals, then almost new. Picture books, he felt, were for children. What he had to say of those pioneer journals may perhaps be explained by the adage, "The shoemaker says there's nothing like leather." The poet, any poet, may be seen (with no reference to his honesty) to be a man of his word: there is nothing, there can be nothing, like words. (Try reading a poem to a medical-school class!) Could

Wordsworth have foreseen television, he would of course have been puzzled and dismayed. So modern and sophisticated a man as Tyrone Guthrie was also rather dismayed. This is how he saw it:

> Those who purvey commercial entertainment know very well that we are all lazy most of the time, and many of us are lazy all the time. Strenuous entertainment does not pay so well as the kind which makes minimal demands upon your faculties. The most paying of all is the kind that can be received with no effort at all, that permits us to take in the entertainment [the instruction?] through the pores of the skin at a level comfortably below consciousness. This is why most Television Entertainment is as it is.[3]

Most television purposes, of course, to be entertainment, and most of it is puerile. There is always (always, one may say hopefully, if insecurely) the glory (when it is glorious, as it so frequently is) of PBS. Many PBS programs expound ideas; sometimes they expound brilliantly, almost always lucidly. Col. Joy's film presentation in Baltimore was a great success as entertainment; it even expounded, or at least presented, an idea or two. One, in fact, was an example of revisionist history. (Assuming the student to be ignorant of the concept in need of revision, he or she would not much require to be disabused of it.) But the entertainment factor certainly predominated. There is no doubt that the visual cortex was occupied. That stuffy old ex-radical, that word-enchanted conservative, William Wordsworth, would doubtless have wanted to know if the mind was occupied too. It is Col. Joy's contention, however, that his course is the sort which is needed for a generation raised on television. Is there, then, to be any difference between an illustrated lecture and a slide show with commentary?

Question and answer, discussion and analysis, follow some USUHS lectures and slide shows, and the essay required at the end of the course in lieu of examination, is presumably pondered from September to tulip time. The library resources are remarkable. The spectrum of different presentations at different levels—some very short, some surprisingly long—includes brief seminars. The opportunity certainly exists for individual mental activity. And yet, the question persists whether full occupation of the visual cortex greatly assists or even to some extent precludes or hinders occupation of the cerebral cortex.

In contrast with the nil challenge of the history of medicine to either of these cortices in the majority of medical schools, the vivid and varied USUHS program must be heartily applauded. Olive drab can sometimes be the liveliest of colors.

Notes

1. Lloyd G. Stevenson, "Putting history to work: some undergraduate essays on the history of medicine," *Journal of the History of Medicine and Allied Sciences,* 1956, *11:* 346–48.

2. Professor Sigerist, Professor Temkin, and others at Johns Hopkins were giving extensively illustrated lectures in the 1930s. The University of Wisconsin has brought together a very extensive collection of medical-history slides, from which other schools, including Johns Hopkins, have obtained some very useful copies. Cf. also James W. Haviland, "Teaching medical history: some unusual aspects," *Bull. Hist. Med.,* 1966, *40:* 168–74. This account of noon-hour history session for first-and-second-year students (students supplying a large part of the material) and evening meetings for fourth-year students, includes a long paragraph (p.173) on the collection, fifteen years ago, of some eight hundred 35 mm color transparencies at the University of Washington, Seattle, "housed in our library, catalogued, and available to anyone."

3. Tyrone Guthrie, "So long as the theater can do miracles," in *Edge of Awareness,* ed. Ned E. Hoopes and Richard Peck (New York: Delacorte Press, 1966), pp. 160–61.

THE TEACHING OF MEDICAL HISTORY BY INSTRUCTORS FROM A VARIETY OF DISCIPLINES*

Alvin E. Rodin and Robert D. Reece

Formal exposure of medical students to the history of their future profession has received variable concern and commitment over the past fifty years. In the last three decades increasing emphasis on the humanities in medical education has resulted in a resurgence of interest in medical history as a curricular activity.

Miller's study of history activities in medical schools in 1968, however, revealed that nineteen out of 105 medical schools had a medical history unit.[1] Regular courses in medical history were given in only ten schools, the number of hours ranging from eight to thirty. In fifteen other schools orientation to medical history was provided by related discussions within various medical courses. There were only five schools in which students took an active role in a seminar format. Only six offered electives in history of medicine, three as a full-time block ranging from one day to two weeks, and three as a part-time informal activity spread over an indefinite period of time. In one, descriptions of patients from the fifteenth to the nineteenth centuries were used as a basis for historical discussions.[2]

The Macy Conference on Education in the History of Medicine, held in 1966, highlighted the fact that neglect of history in medical schools is due to several factors.[3] First, it is difficult to obtain any time in a curriculum already markedly overcrowded with subjects that are directly related to the diagnosis and management of disease. Second, the frequent emphasis on names and dates of individuals and discoveries has failed to interest and stimulate the vast majority of medical students. Third, when medical history is actually placed in the curriculum, the lecture format has been used predominantly, with resultant lack of active student involvement. A fourth factor is that such

*Although Wright State University School of Medicine, Dayton, Ohio, was represented at the symposium in Baltimore in October 1980, this paper was not presented then but was submitted afterwards to the *Bulletin of the History of Medicine*. To keep it in the context of the symposium, it is offered here rather than in the *Bulletin*, the *Bulletin* editor supplying the commentary.

courses often do not have required exams, and are in competititon for students' attention with those that do.

Since Miller's review of 1968, there has been some increase in historical activities in schools of medicine. The majority of students, however, still exhibit little interest in the subject. Instructors are usually trained in history or medicine or both. The discipline of history necessitates documentation, and traditional medicine is concerned with the who, what, and when. These are necessary, but in themselves fail to captivate students. A broader orientation is especially pertinent for the socially conscious students of the past decade. In order to address the above concerns an interdisciplinary and intercollegiate learning experience was developed for students at Wright State University School of Medicine.

An Interdisciplinary Elective

The offering of a two-week elective in history of medicine became possible at Wright State University School of Medicine with the development of a curriculum of seven quarters, each lasting eleven weeks, in the first two years. The elective in the history of medicine was organized for the end of the second quarter of the freshman year, and titled "Orientation To The History of Medicine." The elective was developed to emphasize relationships of medicine with society. Active involvement of students was a major part of the educational design. Three instructors were obtained from medical disciplines and five from fields outside of medicine (table 1).

There were two general goals for this elective. The first was to provide an overall perspective for students undergoing the professionalization process for medical education. The second was to provide sufficient orientation for students to proceed with their own specific areas of historical interest. Major content areas included development of medicine as a profession, development of concepts of health and disease, relationship of medical to nonmedical history, and influence of the nonmedical environment (law, religion, politics, socioeconomics, science, philosophy) on the development of medical concepts and health care delivery systems. The first session was devoted to considerations of possible reasons for the study of the history of medicine, the influence of society on medicine in general, and the development of medicine as a profession. Subsequent sessions were organized on the basis of historical eras. The final two sessions were related to American medicine and medicine in the future.

In order to develop a relevant focus and to help organize the large

TABLE 1. Outline of Two-week Elective on Orientation to the History of Medicine

MAJOR CONTENT AREA	MAJOR EMPHASIS	STUDENT TOPIC POSITION	DISCIPLINE OF INSTRUCTOR
The History of Medicine	Why study the history of medicine		Religion
Society and Medicine	Influence of society on medicine		Sociology
Physicians in History	Development of medicine as a profession		Medical Education
Primitive Medicine	Relationships between magic, religion, and science	The Medicine Man was effective	Anthropology
Greco-Roman Medicine	Influence of philosophy on medical concepts	The Hippocratic Oath is outmoded	Classics
Medieval Medicine	Medical knowledge as absolute truth	The Church inhibited medical progress	History
Renaissance Medicine	Characteristics of supposition and observation	The Rise of Science decreased humanism	Philosophy
Seventeenth-to-Nineteenth-Century Medicine	Influence of disease concepts on medical practice	Physicians did more harm than good	History
Twentieth-Century Medicine	Consequences of the experimental method	Technology is the basis for medical progress	Pharmacology
American Medicine	Types of medical systems	Private Medical Practice provides the best care	Medical Education
Future Medicine	The future in the past	Patient-Doctor Relationship will decrease	Medical Education

amount of material, two statements were developed for each historical era. One was an area of major emphasis for orientation of group discussions and reading assignments. The other was a controversial statement of a position to be taken in the individual student presentation.

Each segment was organized on a similar basis. The first activity was a half-hour presentation by the instructor on the area, followed by student discussion. Students were then given specific reading assignments in preparation for continuation of the discussion the next day. One student was assigned an individual project based on the position statement for the area. The following day the student gave a ten-minute presentation on his project. This was followed by student discussion in general. Up to one and a half hours were then spent in general group discussion on the historical era, with the instructor acting as the discussion leader. Only one of the instructors, who was also the chairman of the elective, was an M.D. The remainder held doctorates in other disciplines.

The elective was chosen by nine freshmen medical students out of a class of thirty-two. It was one of six electives offered at this time. All students attended each of the scheduled periods, which consisted of ten morning sessions of three hours each. Each student submitted a written report on his individual project. Students used a variety of resources in assembling their accounts. Books relating to the elective were available on reserve at the Health Science Library. Some students obtained reference material from the general university library. Others discussed their topic individually with instructors.

In evaluation of the elective, students gave the session on future medicine the highest rating for overall interest, and the group discussion and individual projects the highest rating for teaching/learning formats. These ratings were reinforced by written comments of students. They emphasized the value of having instructors from various nonmedical disciplines and the importance of the extensive student participation. Suggestions included providing audio-visual aids such as maps, slides, and movies, and improving the quality of some of the reading assignments.

Discussion

This interdisciplinary and intercollegiate elective in the history of medicine met the pedagogic objectives in teaching the history of medicine as enunciated by George Rosen at the Macy Foundation conference of 1966.[4] His first objective was to show the development of medicine as a whole by emphasizing continuity in time and recurrent elements. This was met by having sessions on the influence of society on medicine and the professionalization process at the beginning, and by ending the elective with consideration of the future of medicine on the basis of the past. Common elements considered in the various historical eras included philosophical and socioeconomic influences on medicine.

Rosen's second objective was to deal with the problem of changing medicine by analyzing changes in the past and recognizing forces that have shaped medicine so that the student may in some degree be prepared for changes which will continue to occur. This objective is quite similar to the content areas enunciated for the elective period. Objective number three was to lay bare the origins of medical ideas and values and their role and significance, and to show how the translation of medical values into policies is historically conditioned. This was accomplished by consideration of the philosophical and political orientation of each historical era and their influence on health care delivery as well as on medical discoveries.

Rosen's fourth objective related to showing students that knowledge in one medical discipline is of value in comprehending apparently unrelated developments in other branches. The elective went even further by showing the relationship of the evolution of medicine to other areas of human endeavor, and, in illustration of the points, featuring instructors from nonmedical disciplines.

Objective number five was to develop a sense of historical perspective and thus a salutary critical point of view towards fads and modish trends in medicine. This was addressed in particular in the segment on American medicine which considered in depth various systems of medicine, such as homeopathy, and various fads such as spurious cures for cancer.

It is not possible to determine any specific attitudinal changes on the part of the students who were involved in the elective. Even if some of them do engage in medical historical activities in the future, such an orientation may have been present before the elective. Possibly the most significant outcome is that a two-week exposure to the history of medicine obtained and maintained the interest and enthusiasm of medical students throughout with consequent high ratings. Another benefit, which cannot be documented aside from narrative, consists of statements by instructors that they obtained valuable insights from working with instructors from other disciplines.

Notes

1. G. Miller, "The teaching of medical history in the United States and Canada: report of a field survey," *Bull. Hist. Med.*, 1969, *43*: 259–67.

2. A. E. Rodin and A. J. Strano, "Case-oriented presentation of medical history: the D.E.A.D. conference," *J. Med. Educ.*, 1967, *42*: 886–91.

3. J. B. Blake, ed., *Education in the History of Medicine*, Report of Macy Conference, 22–24 June 1966 (New York: Hafner Publishing, 1968).

4. G. Rosen, "What medical history should be taught to medical students?" in Blake, *Education in the History of Medicine*, pp. 21–22.

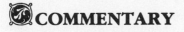

COMMENTARY

Lloyd G. Stevenson

In the seventy years since the Flexner Report, American medical education has undergone many changes, but in the thirty-five years since World War II it has hardly turned away from the mirror; its anxious self-examination may even be said to have had a certain teenager quality and certainly it has discovered blemishes more serious than blackheads. To correct its shortcomings it has revised and re-revised the curriculum. In some centers a new plan has not been allowed to take effect fully before it has been supplanted by one still newer. Not all of the innovations, of course, have been substantially new; a few have reintroduced practices of the eighteenth or of a yet earlier century. With the encouragement of the Commonwealth Fund the curriculum planners have worked hard, but the patterns they have produced have come to seem more and more familiar. One of the most vital of all transformations (whether new or old) has been increased emphasis on the role of the student: one midwestern university announced the "discovery" of the student in 1950. Another frequently announced realization has been that of the value of the humanities in medical education. This has led, in certain instances, to a resurgence of interest in medical history, in others to a minestrone (the word means something served) containing history, sociology, anthropology, philosophy, and possibly bits of pasta. But valuable integrated efforts have no doubt been achieved and Wright State's would appear to be one of them; this may be in part because, in Dayton, the history of medicine has been menstruum and not merely one of many ingredients.

If the late Professor George Rosen—whose aims for the history of medicine, as expressed in 1966, have been taken as the standard against which to measure Dayton's success—did not himself organize and take part in teaching programs involving several of his colleagues from various departments, this, one assumes, was because of the wide range of his learning, his interests, and his achievement. His example—and the range of the claims and the proposals put forward during this symposium—suggest, of course, that there is more than one way to attain the goals and more than one opinion of what they should be.

But if successes of several kinds have been described, the day has also heard a few admissions of difficulty and even of unsuccess. Modification of the pattern is called for. The general renovations of medical schools that have characterized recent decades and that have been aimed at the improvement of all areas, preclinical and clinical, have often included provision for more student participation, for multidisciplinary teaching, and for block-time electives. To put these three elements of pedagogic reform together in the teaching of medical history is at least relatively novel, and perhaps absolutely so.

In Miller's study of medical-history activities in medical schools in 1968, only five schools were found in which students took an active role in a seminar format. That students can take an intelligent part in the discussion of themes that they have not previously encountered was recently questioned by Temkin. The answer that assigned readings will supply the basis is surely something of a brush-off unless it can be assumed that a genuine teaching seminar is to be operated—and such seminars have usually succeeded only at a graduate level. This is not to say that they cannot succeed in medical schools, for it has been done for other purposes.

Multidisciplinary teaching, warmly advocated by Case-Western Reserve and by many other innovating centers, is ordinarily thought of as sustaining rather than replacing the teaching of a particular area in the curriculum. The internist has not been displaced by an assortment of his colleagues from the medical sciences, far less by an array of physicists, chemists, and mathematicians from another corner of the campus or even from another campus. Medical history, however, belongs with the support troops, and since it is related in obvious ways to various departments throughout the university, there is an administrative temptation to let a group of them take its place. Who, it might be asked, cannot teach medical history?

Many courses in medical history begin, as they do in Dayton, on the defensive: Why study the history of medicine? It perhaps is logical, then, to begin—as they do in Dayton but rarely elsewhere—with an instructor from Religion, presumably one skilled in apologetics. The later sequence is similarly reasonable—primitive medicine (Anthropology), Greek and Roman medicine (Classics), Medieval medicine (History), Renaissance medicine (Philosophy) and so forth. A little less apparent is the reason for Medical Education to undertake the responsibility for "Types of medical systems." This seems to mean systems of medical-care financing, since the Student Topic Position is given in this ringing declaration: "Private Medical Practice provides the best care." Medical Education also looks after "Future Medicine," reported to be the most popular segment of the course, and one on which the student position is: "Patient-Doctor Relationship will decrease." A broader orientation than the conventional one, we are told at the beginning of the paper, is "especially pertinent for the socially conscious student of the past decade." The student conception of relevance gradually emerges.

How the Student Topic Position was arrived at is not stated. Did the students start or finish with such views as these: "The Medicine Man was effective," "The Hippocratic Oath is outmoded" and, from the seventeenth century to the nineteenth century, "Physicians did more harm than good"? We take it that each of these was a position (or resolution) adopted for the purposes of a three-hour debate—or at any rate a discussion. Was the conclusion of each meeting a judgment passed on, for example, the primitives, the Greeks, the medieval church ("The Church inhibited medical progress")? The student position, as listed, was not, of course, necessarily sustained. It may often have been overturned. Or perhaps—and this, of course, is more probable—no categorical conclusion was reached. May it be assumed, however, that the "issues" were thoroughly aired? May it be assumed that they were the right issues on which to spend half a day, for each, and that they arose from (rather than being imposed upon) the ascertainable facts? The initial doubt that historical facts are worth ascertaining—at least in medicine's past—beclouds the question. It is clear that the course in Dayton picks up speed and interest as it advances and that it zooms through the present and into the future with something like a cheer. And yet the future is anchored, so it seems, in the past.

If a brief statement of the Wright State system and a one-page outline of the course can evoke such a flood of doubts, objections, and queries, it seems probable that the program itself has given rise to spirited participation. The opportunity for this has presumably been unusually great because of the generous time blocks, few though they are. It is curious that the sketch and outline provided give the impression, somehow, of a once-over-lightly. Is vigorous participation proof of effectiveness? Most centers would be more than happy if they could claim it. Spirited participation may be inspired, or at any rate suggested, by a Socrates—and also by a pornographic movie.

At least two of the other teaching programs described in the course of this symposium—one in Texas and one in Florida—line up a considerable variety of disciplines. Harvard has declared in print the variability of its approach and the number of departments it is able to enlist. McGill has recently changed the name of a department originally aimed at medical history in such a way as to suggest that the department will henceforth devote itself to humanities and social sciences very broadly indeed: much in the manner in which the same school (like many others in the nineteenth century and earlier) taught a whole range of medical sciences under the rubric of "The Institutes of Medicine." Another cluster in old curricula used to be, not infrequently, medical ethics and medical jurisprudence. Medical ethics, at least, may now be spliced into the medical humanities and social sciences, somewhere in the region which once bore the name history. Perhaps the message of Galveston, Montreal, Cambridge, and Dayton is that history is all right provided it teaches good ethics, good economics, and whatever other goods need teaching. To teach history as history would (surely?) be mere antiquarianism. History, however, may serve to remind us that this was once medicine's attitude to science. Well enough, science, if directly subservient to bedside medicine; pursued for its own sake it was often considered "curious" but unimportant.

It is possible (is it also probable?) that a new generation will revel in a new edition of the "Institutes," one composed of all the varied elements of medical education that are now generally made known by their absence. Whatever the label and whatever the mix, the Wright-State-style course seems to succeed on its own terms and to be well liked and rewarding. Rewarding, that is, for the comparative few who elect to take it. Could it be that they constitute that segment of the class needing it the least—the segment most likely to find a way out of the wilderness unassisted?

In one sure way, recalling the nineteenth-century habit of leaving instruction in pharmacology (to take one example) to a practitioner of medicine, the Dayton plan looks back to the past: it absolves the university from the necessity of hiring a medical historian. And is that not in the spirit of the nineteen-eighties?

🕮 LIST OF CONTRIBUTORS

Edward C. Atwater, M.A., M.D.
University of Rochester
Rochester, New York 14620

Don G. Bates, M.D., Ph.D.
McGill University
Montreal, Quebec, Canada H3G 1Y6

Gert H. Brieger, M.D., Ph.D.
University of California-San Francisco
San Francisco, California 94143

Chester R. Burns, M.D., Ph.D.
University of Texas Medical Branch
Galveston, Texas 77550

Jerome J. Bylebyl, Ph.D.
The Johns Hopkins University
Baltimore, Maryland 21205

John K. Crellin, M.D., Ph.D.
Duke University Medical Center
Durham, North Carolina 27710

Robert P. Hudson, M.A., M.D.
University of Kansas Medical Center
Kansas City, Kansas 66103

Saul Jarcho, M.D.
11 W. 69th Street
New York, New York 10023

Robert J. T. Joy, M.D.
Uniformed Services University of the Health Sciences
Bethesda, Maryland 20014

Russell C. Maulitz, M.D., Ph.D.
University of Pennsylvania
Philadelphia, Pennsylvania 19104

Pauline M. H. Mazumdar, M.B., B.Ch., Ph.D.
University of Toronto
Toronto, Ontario, Canada M5S 1A1

John Parascandola, Ph.D.
University of Wisconsin
Madison, Wisconsin 53706

Robert D. Reece, Ph.D.
Wright State University
Dayton, Ohio 45401

Guenter Risse, M.D., Ph.D.
University of Wisconsin
Madison, Wisconsin 53706

Alvin E. Rodin, M.D.
Wright State University
Dayton, Ohio 45401

Barbara G. Rosenkrantz, Ph.D.
Harvard University
Cambridge, Massachusetts 02138

Todd L. Savitt, Ph.D.
University of Florida
Gainesville, Florida 32610

Lloyd G. Stevenson, M.D., Ph.D.
The Johns Hopkins University
Baltimore, Maryland 21205

Arthur Viseltear, Ph.D.
Yale University
New Haven, Connecticut 06510